RECOVER
with
GAPS

RECOVER
with
GAPS

A Cookbook of 101 Healthy and Easy Recipes That I Used to
Heal My ULCERATIVE COLITIS while ON THE GAPS DIET.
Heal Your Gut Too!

Pamela Jenkins
&
Donna Gates

Paperback ISBN:
ISBN-13: 978-1502873873
ISBN-10: 1502873877

DISCLAIMER

The information provided in this book is for educational purposes only. I am not a physician and this is not to be taken as medical advice or a recommendation to stop eating other foods. The information provided in this book is based on experiences and interpretations of past and current research available. You should consult your doctor to ensure that the recipes in this book are appropriate for your individual circumstances. If you have any health issues or pre-existing conditions, please consult your doctor before implementing any of the information that is presented in this cookbook. Results may vary from individual to individual. Mention of specific companies, entities, organizations or authorities in this book does not imply endorsement by the author or publisher, nor does mention of specific companies, entities, organizations, or authorities imply that they endorse this book, its author, or the publisher. This book is for informational purposes only and the author does not accept any responsibilities for any liabilities or damages, real or perceived, resulting from the use of this resource.

Table of Contents

I HEALED MY LEAKY GUT— YOU CAN TOO!

"I have found that food is an extremely powerful way of dealing with disease—the most powerful way. Many people don't realize how powerful food is."
—Dr Natasha Campbell-McBride MD, creator and author of
Gut & Psychology Syndrome (GAPS)

Now you can really heal your gut. It's about time! If you are hurting because of this challenge, then, I know exactly how you might feel. For me, my suffering wasn't much different. "I can't take this any longer!" That's what I thought to myself as I tried to endure another night of wrenching abdominal pain which kept me from sleeping. Ulcerative colitis was literally my biggest nightmare. Yes, I had been to several doctors. Yes, I had done several tests. Yes, I had been taking different prescription drugs. But all was to no avail in healing me from the terror of ulcerative colitis. As my condition worsened, I became worried about being hooked to prescription drugs for merely symptom relief. Besides, after all that, the problem was still there. I was desperate for help.

As I became more desperate, I also became more aggressive. I started to look everywhere I could for help. One day as I browsed the internet, I discovered this life-changing diet. I listened to author, Dr Natasha Campbell-McBride talking about her book, *Gut and Psychology Syndrome GAPS* and her diet concept in an interview with Dr. Mercola. It wasn't long before I got the feeling that she was talking directly to me as she pointed out how the health of the gut affects the rest of the body. As I listened to her, I became hopeful that this was possibly the answer I've been looking for. There's no way I could go on without giving this diet a try. I am happy that I got results with the GAPS Diet. Fortunately, I healed my gut and it changed my life—not just my health.

If you've not yet read her life-changing book, I urge you to do so. Like me, in the end you'll be empowered to turn your health situation around. Now, I am not going to get into what the diet is all about. Instead, in my cookbook, I am sharing my personal "go-to" recipes which I've used to successfully follow the GAPS Diet and have gotten great results.

It is true that adapting to a new diet can be a daunting task, and for this reason, new recipe ideas are always helpful. This cookbook was created to make your journey on this diet even easier. Based on my own experience, one of my greatest challenges was to prepare a variety of meals based on the ingredients allowed. Consequently, in this cookbook I am sharing a compilation of some of my own creative recipes based on the GAPS Diet guidelines.

I encourage you today to start restoring the health of your gut. So, whether you're experiencing allergies, food intolerance, autism or other digestive disorders, there is hope. My best relief from ulcerative colitis came after I tried the GAPS Diet. I hope that you'll enjoy these recipes. However, even more importantly, I hope you find these recipes to be useful on your journey to restore your health, lose weight, or to simply heal your gut.

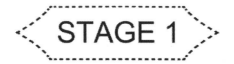

Homemade Fish Broth

This homemade fish broth is quite easy and provides a magnificent base for fish soups, chowders, seafood risotto, as well as many more dishes.

Servings: 4
Prep Time: 10 minutes
Cooking Time: 1 hour 30 minutes

Ingredients:

2 medium-sized whole Sole Fish
12 cups Purified Water
Natural unprocessed Salt, to taste
Freshly Crushed Black Pepper, to taste

Directions:

1. Remove the meat from the fish. In a large soup pan, add the heads, bones, fins, skin and tail to the water. Bring to boiling point on a high heat.
2. Reduce the heat and simmer for 1 to 1½ hours.
3. Stir in the salt and pepper in the last 10 minutes. Strain through a strainer lined with cheesecloth.
4. Transfer to a sterilized food container to store until required.

***Note Well:** In order to make other broths, simply replace the fish in the above recipe with any of the following: fish bones, fish heads, fish fins or other inexpensive fish cuttings. Be mindful of adjusting the cooking time when necessary.*

Home-style Chicken Broth

There is nothing quite like the deep rich flavor, and the golden color of homemade chicken stock. This stock provides amazing flavors for chicken soups, stews and even for rice dishes.

Servings: 4
Prep Time: 10 minutes
Cooking Time: 3 hours

Ingredients:

3 pounds Organic Whole Chicken
16 cups Purified Water
Natural unprocessed Salt, to taste
Freshly Crushed Black Pepper, to taste

Directions:

1. Cut the chicken in half, lengthways, and place in a large soup pan with the water, salt and black pepper. Bring to boiling point on a high heat.
2. Reduce the heat and simmer for 2½ to 3 hours.
3. Strain the broth through a strainer lined with a cheesecloth.
4. Transfer to a sterilized food container and store until required.

Note Well: *In order to make other broths, simply replace the meat in the above recipe with any of the following meats: duck, goose, whole pigeons, giblets from chicken, pheasants or other low-cost meats. Be mindful of adjusting the cooking time based on the type of meat chosen.*

Shredded Chicken Soup

This is a great soup recipe. The combination of chicken and carrots makes this a tasty dish, made with homemade broth. Garnish with freshly chopped cilantro.

Servings: 4
Prep Time: 10 minutes
Cooking Time: 30 minutes

Ingredients:

6 cups Homemade Chicken Broth
1 small Onion, chopped finely
2 medium Carrots, peeled and chopped
2 Garlic Cloves, chopped
2 cups shredded, cooked, boneless Organic Chicken
1 Scallion, chopped
Natural unprocessed Salt, to taste
Freshly Crushed Black Pepper, to taste

Directions:

1. In a large soup pan, add the broth and bring to boiling point on a medium-high heat. Add the onion, carrot and garlic to the pan.
2. Reduce the heat, cover, and simmer for 15 to 20 minutes.
3. Stir in the chicken, scallion, salt and black pepper. Simmer for a further 10 minutes before serving.

Florets Chicken Soup

This soup is easy to make and quickly prepared. This blended and smooth vegetable soup is really good for a comforting meal, and tastes delicious.

Servings: 4
Prep Time: 15 minutes
Cooking Time: 23 minutes

Ingredients:

6 cups Homemade Chicken Broth
1 medium Onion, chopped
2 cups Carrots, peeled and chopped
2 Garlic Cloves, chopped
2 cups Broccoli Florets, chopped roughly
Natural unprocessed Salt, to taste
Freshly Crushed Black Pepper, to taste

Directions:

1. In a large soup pan, add the broth and bring to boiling point on a medium-high heat. Add the onion, carrot and garlic to the pan.
2. Reduce the heat, cover, and simmer for 10 to 15 minutes.
3. Add the broccoli and simmer for an additional 5 minutes. Remove from the heat and cool slightly. Transfer the soup into a blender and pulse until smooth.
4. Return the soup to the pan and cook for a further 2 to 3 minutes. Season with salt and black pepper before serving.
5.

Mixed Yellow Soup

This is a filling, delicious soup that your whole family will love! This extremely easy to make soup can also be made on a tight budget.

Servings: 4
Prep Time: 15 minutes
Cooking Time: 23 minutes

Ingredients:

6 cups Homemade Chicken Broth
1 small Onion, chopped
3 Garlic Cloves, minced
3 cups Cauliflower Florets, chopped roughly
1½ cups Carrots, peeled and chopped
1 pound Fresh Yellow Tuna, cubed
Natural unprocessed Salt, to taste
Freshly Crushed Black Pepper, to taste

Directions:

1. In a large soup pan, add the broth and bring to boiling point on a medium-high heat. Add the onion, garlic, cauliflower, carrot and tuna.
2. Reduce the heat, cover, and simmer for 20 minutes.
3. Remove from the heat and cool slightly. Transfer the soup into a blender and pulse until smooth.
4. Return the soup into the pan and cook for a further 2 to 3 minutes. Season with salt and black pepper before serving.

Cauliflower Twist Soup

This soup is filled with chunks of chicken, cauliflower and carrot. This dish is really delicious, easy to make, and is healthy as well.

Servings: 4
Prep Time: 15 minutes
Cooking Time: 25 minutes

Ingredients:

6 cups Homemade Chicken Broth
2 cups boneless Organic Chicken, in bite-sized pieces
1 small Onion, chopped
3 Carrots, peeled and chopped
3 Garlic Cloves, minced
3 cups Cauliflower Florets, chopped roughly
Natural unprocessed Salt, to taste
Freshly Crushed Black Pepper, to taste

Directions:

1. In a large soup pan, add the broth and chicken, and bring to boiling point on a high heat. Reduce the heat, cover, and simmer for 8 to 10 minutes.
2. Add the onion, carrot, garlic and cauliflower, and bring to boiling point again.
3. Reduce the heat, cover, and simmer for a further 10 to 15 minutes.
4. Season with salt and black pepper before serving.

Picaso Soup

This is one of the best and healthiest soups. It will be great starter for a main meal, as well as being perfect for a dinner on a cold winter's night.

Servings: 4
Prep Time: 15 minutes
Cooking Time: 23 minutes

Ingredients:

6 cups Homemade Chicken Broth
1 small Onion, chopped
2 Scallions, chopped
4 Garlic Cloves, minced
5 cups Cauliflower Florets, chopped roughly
Natural unprocessed Salt, to taste
Freshly Crushed Black Pepper, to taste

Directions:

1. In a large soup pan, add the broth and bring to boiling point on a medium-high heat. Add the onion, scallion, garlic and cauliflower.
2. Reduce the heat, cover, and simmer for 20 minutes.
3. Remove from heat and cool slightly. Transfer the soup into a blender and pulse until smooth and creamy.
4. Return the soup into the pan and cook for a further 2 to 3 minutes. Season with salt and black pepper before serving.

Tomato Chi Soup

This is a mildly flavored tomato and zucchini soup which has tender pieces of cod. This soup is appropriate for all stages of the diet.

Servings: 4
Prep Time: 15 minutes
Cooking Time: 20 minutes

Ingredients:

6 cups Homemade Fish Broth
1 pound boneless Cod Fillets, chopped
1 small Onion, chopped
4 Garlic Cloves, minced
3 Tomatoes, seeded and chopped
2 Zucchinis, peeled, seeded and chopped
Natural unprocessed Salt, to taste
Freshly Crushed Black Pepper, to taste

Directions:

1. In a large soup pan, add the broth and bring to boiling point on a medium-high heat. Add the fish, onion, garlic, tomatoes and zucchini.
2. Reduce the heat, cover, and simmer for 15 to 20 minutes.
3. Season with salt and black pepper before serving.

Mixed Squash Soup

This creamy, pureed vegetable soup is not only super simple and nourishing, but also a nice way to make a nourishing and tasty soup.

Servings: 4
Prep Time: 15 minutes
Cooking Time: 28 minutes

Ingredients:

5 cups Homemade Chicken Broth
5 cups mixed Squashes (Butternut Squash, Winter Squash, Yellow Squash) - peeled, seeded and chopped
1 large Onion, chopped
1-inch fresh Ginger, peeled and chopped finely
5 Garlic Cloves, chopped
Natural unprocessed Salt, to taste
Freshly Crushed Black Pepper, to taste

Directions:

1. In a large soup pan, add the broth and bring to boiling point on a medium-high heat. Add the squashes, onion, ginger and garlic.
2. Reduce the heat, cover, and simmer for 20 to 25 minutes.
3. Remove from the heat and cool slightly. Transfer the soup into a blender and pulse until smooth and creamy.
4. Return the soup into the pan and cook for a further 2 to 3 minutes. Season with salt and black pepper before serving.

Gingery Carrot Soup

This amazing soup will be a great addition to your menu list.

Servings: 4
Prep Time: 15 minutes
Cooking Time: 20 minutes

Ingredients:

6 cups Homemade Chicken Broth
2 medium Onions, chopped
1-inch fresh Ginger, peeled and chopped finely
4 cups Carrots, peeled and chopped
Natural unprocessed Salt, to taste
Freshly Crushed Black Pepper, to taste

Directions:

1. In a large soup pan, add the broth and bring to boiling point on a medium-high heat. Add the onion, ginger and carrots.
2. Reduce the heat, cover, and simmer for 10 to 15 minutes.
3. Remove from the heat and cool slightly. Transfer the soup into a blender and pulse until smooth and creamy.
4. Return the soup into the pan and cook for 2 to 3 minutes. Season with salt and black pepper before serving.

Kale Combo

This is a hearty and filling soup recipe. This dish is perfect for easy weeknight dinners during the autumn and winter.

Servings: 4
Prep Time: 10 minutes
Cooking Time: 20 minutes

Ingredients:

6 cups Homemade Chicken Broth
2 cups shredded, cooked, boneless Organic Chicken
4 cups fresh Kale, trimmed and chopped
Natural unprocessed Salt, to taste
Freshly Crushed Black Pepper, to taste

Directions:

1. In a large soup pan, add the broth and bring to boiling point on a medium-high heat. Add the chicken and kale to the pan.
2. Reduce the heat, cover, and simmer for 15 to 20 minutes.
3. Season with salt and black pepper before serving.

Spinach Dip Soup

This soup is creamy and has a velvety texture.

Servings: 4
Prep Time: 10 minutes
Cooking Time: 28 minutes

Ingredients:

6 cups Homemade Chicken Broth
1 Onion, chopped
3 Garlic Cloves, minced
3 cups Cauliflower Florets, chopped finely
3 cups fresh Spinach, trimmed and chopped
Natural unprocessed Salt, to taste
Freshly Crushed Black Pepper, to taste

Directions:

1. In a large soup pan, add the broth and bring to boiling point on a medium-high heat. Add the onion, garlic and cauliflower.
2. Reduce the heat, cover, and simmer for 15 minutes. Stir in the spinach and simmer for an additional 10 minutes.
3. Remove from the heat and cool slightly. Transfer the soup into a blender and pulse until smooth and creamy.
4. Return the soup into the pan and cook for 2 to 3 minutes. Season with salt and black pepper before serving.

Homemade Kefir

Kefir is like yogurt, but it is easier to make, and of course healthier! If you have not tasted Kefir before, you'll find yourself loving this.

Servings: 4
Prep Time: 2 days

Ingredients:
1 tablespoon Kefir Grains
4 cups Organic Milk

Directions:
1. Place the kefir into a sterilized glass jar. Pour the milk over the kefir grains.
2. Cover tightly and keep at room temperature for 1 to 2 days, stirring with a plastic spoon periodically.
3. Strain the kefir and refrigerate.

Home-style Yogurt

Yogurt is still one of the best foods for delivering probiotics to your body. There's much assurance and satisfaction of making it for yourself. It is also a much healthier and cheaper alternative than getting the store bought yogurt.

Servings: 4
Prep Time: 10 minutes (plus 10-13 hours for fermentation and refrigeration)
Cooking Time: 5-6 minutes

Ingredients:
4 cups Pasteurized Whole Milk
1½ teaspoons Unflavored Gelatin
1 Yogurt Starter Packet

Directions:
1. In a pan, add milk on medium-high heat. Heat, stirring continuously until it reaches to the temperature of 165 degrees F. Remove from heat and let it cool until the temperature reaches to 110 degrees F.
2. Add gelatin and stir until well combined. Add yogurt starter and stir well.
3. Transfer the milk into a dry jar. Cover and place in a slightly warm place for 8 to 10 hours.
4. Place in the refrigerator in order to chill the yogurt for at least 3 hours before serving.

Homemade Sauerkraut

Historically, because of its high vitamin C content, sauerkraut was very useful in keeping you healthy throughout the winter months when no fresh food was available. Sauerkraut is great for all phases where it can be tolerated.

Servings: 4
Prep Time: 30 minutes (Plus time to "sit")

Ingredients:
1 medium Head Cabbage, shredded
1 teaspoon Caraway Seeds
1½ teaspoons natural unprocessed Salt
1 cup Filtered Water

Directions:
1. In a large bowl, combine the cabbage, caraway seeds and salt. Set aside for 10 to 20 minutes.
2. Transfer the cabbage mixture into a sterilized jar and compress the cabbage. Pour water over the cabbage and seal with a lid.
3. Store the jar for 2 to 3 weeks at 65 - 75 degrees F.
4. Transfer the sauerkraut into small sterilized jars and refrigerate.

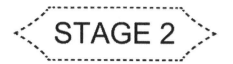

Munchy Chicken Stew

This brightly tasting and delicious stew recipe is packed with healthy vitamins. Garnish with freshly chopped scallions.

Servings: 4
Prep Time: 10 minutes
Cooking Time: 1 hour 6 minutes

Ingredients:

2 tablespoons Ghee
1 pound diced, boneless, Organic Chicken Breast
1 small Onion, chopped finely
1 teaspoon Garlic, minced
½ tablespoon finely diced fresh Ginger Root
2 cups Carrots, peeled and cut into wedges
1 cup small Turnips, peeled and cut into wedges
3 tablespoons fresh Basil, chopped
1 cup Homemade Chicken Broth
Natural unprocessed Salt, to taste

Directions:

1. In a large pan, melt the ghee on a medium-high heat. For 4 to 5 minutes sauté the chicken, or cook until browned. Transfer the chicken into a bowl.
2. In the same pan, add the onion and sauté for 4 to 5 minutes. Add the garlic and ginger, and sauté for 1 minute more. Add the carrot and turnip, and sauté for 5 minutes. Add the chicken, salt, basil and broth. Bring the pan to the boil.
3. Reduce the heat to low. Cover and simmer for 35 to 45

4. minutes.

Spaghetti Thigh Stew

This recipe makes a nutritious, filling stew which not only tastes delicious, but is also great for a simple meal. Top with fresh cilantro leaves.

Servings: 4
Prep Time: 15 minutes
Cooking Time: 51 minutes

Ingredients:
2 tablespoons Ghee
1 pound de-boned Organic Chicken Thighs
1 small Onion, chopped finely
2 Garlic Cloves, minced
1 cup Homemade Chicken Broth
½ cup Grape Tomatoes, seeded and halved
1 teaspoon fresh Basil, chopped
1 teaspoon fresh Thyme, chopped
4 cups diced Spaghetti Squash, peeled and seeded
Natural unprocessed Salt, to taste

Directions:
1. In a large pan, melt the ghee on a medium-high heat. For 4 to 5 minutes sauté the chicken, or cook until browned on both sides. Transfer the chicken into a bowl.
2. In the same pan, add the onion and sauté for 4 to 5 minutes. Add the garlic and sauté for 1 minute more. Add the chicken, broth, tomatoes, basil, thyme and salt, and bring to boiling point.
3. Reduce the heat to low. Cover and simmer for 15 to 20 minutes. Stir in the squash. Cover and simmer for a further 15 to 20 minutes.
4. Serve hot.

31

Lamb Shoulder Stew

This healthy recipe makes a hearty meal that will be particularly enjoyed by all the family. This thick, filling stew is usually served with a topping of fresh parsley leaves.

Servings: 4
Prep Time: 15 minutes
Cooking Time: 2 hours 11 minutes

Ingredients:

2 tablespoons Ghee
1 pound diced, boneless, Organic Lamb Shoulder
1 small Onion, chopped finely
1 Garlic Clove, minced
½ cup Plum Tomatoes, skinned, seeded and chopped very finely
1 teaspoon finely diced fresh Parsley Leaves
1½ cups Homemade Chicken Broth
Natural unprocessed Salt, to taste

Directions:

1. In a large pan, melt the ghee on a medium-high heat. Cook the lamb for 5 minutes, or until completely browned. Transfer the lamb into a bowl.
2. In the same pan, add the onion and sauté for 4 to 5 minutes. Add the garlic and sauté for 1 minute more. Add the lamb, tomatoes, parsley, broth, and salt, and bring to boiling point.
3. Reduce the heat to low. Cover and simmer for 1½ to 2 hours.

Weekend Beef Stew

This is one of the most flavorful and aromatic beef stews. Each bite of this stew has a nice strong kick of fresh herbs. Garnish with chopped fresh cilantro.

Servings: 4
Prep Time: 15 minutes
Cooking Time: 2 hours 25 minutes

Ingredients:

2 tablespoons Ghee
1 pound Organic Lean Beef, cut into chunks
Natural unprocessed Salt, to taste
1 small Onion, chopped finely
2 Garlic Cloves, minced
2 Plum Tomatoes, skinned, seeded and chopped very finely
3 Carrots, peeled and diced
2 tablespoons diced fresh Thyme Leaves
2 tablespoons diced fresh Rosemary Leaves
3 cups Homemade Chicken Broth

Directions:

1. In a large pan, melt the ghee on a medium-high heat. Add the beef and sprinkle with salt. Cook for 5 to 6 minutes per side. Transfer the beef into a bowl.
2. In the same pan, add the onion and sauté for 4 to 5 minutes. Add the garlic and sauté for 1 minute more. Add the tomatoes and sauté for about 3 minutes. Add the carrots and sauté for an additional 5 minutes.
3. Add the beef, broth and fresh herbs to the pan. Bring to boiling point before reducing the heat to medium-low. Simmer the covered pot, stirring occasionally, for approximately 1½ to 2 hours.
4. Season with salt and serve immediately.

Rosemary Stew Cod

Treat your family and guests with this great dish. This fish stew is delicious and simple to prepare. Garnish with freshly chopped rosemary.

Servings: 4
Prep Time: 15 minutes
Cooking Time: 23 minutes

Ingredients:

1 tablespoon Ghee
½ cup Onion, chopped finely
1 Garlic Clove, minced
2 cups Tomatoes, skinned, seeded and chopped very finely
1 tablespoon fresh Dill, chopped
1 tablespoon fresh Thyme, chopped
1 tablespoon fresh Rosemary, chopped
1¼ cups Homemade Fish Broth
1 pound Cod Fillets, cut into 1½-inch pieces
Natural unprocessed Salt, to taste

Directions:

1. In a large skillet, melt the ghee on a medium heat. Sauté the onion and garlic for 4 to 5 minutes. Add the tomatoes and fresh herbs, and sauté for 2 to 3 minutes.
2. Add the broth to the skillet. Bring to boiling before reducing the heat. Simmer, covered, for 8 to 10 minutes.
3. Stir in the fish and return to the boil. Reduce the heat, cover, and simmer for 4 to 5 minutes.
4. Season with salt and serve hot.

Roma Casserole

The combination of vegetables used in this casserole makes this dish delicious. This casserole is wonderfully flavored and simple to make.

Servings: 4
Prep Time: 15 minutes
Cooking Time: 50 minutes

Ingredients:

1 pound cubed, boneless, Organic Chicken Breast
2 tablespoons Ghee, melted and divided
3 tablespoons Homemade Chicken Broth
Natural unprocessed Salt, to taste
3 Zucchinis, peeled, seeded and cut into bite size pieces
¼ cup Roma Tomatoes, seeded and cubed
¼ cup fresh Rosemary, chopped

Directions:

1. Preheat the oven to 350 degrees F and lightly grease a casserole dish.
2. In a large pan, heat 1 tablespoon of the ghee on a medium-high heat. Sauté the chicken for 5 minutes, or until completely browned. Transfer the chicken into the prepared casserole dish. Pour the broth over the chicken and sprinkle with salt.
3. Place the zucchini and tomato over the chicken. Sprinkle with chopped rosemary and drizzle with the remaining melted ghee.
4. Bake for about 45 minutes.

Yellow Meatballs Casserole

This is a healthy and tasty twist on meatballs and squash that your entire family will devour! The fresh herbs used in making the meatballs provide a nice "kick" to this meal.

Servings: 4
Prep Time: 15 minutes
Cooking Time: 45 minutes

Ingredients:
1 pound Organic Ground Beef
1 tablespoon fresh Cilantro, minced
1 tablespoon fresh Mint, minced
2 Garlic Cloves, minced
1 large diced Yellow Squash, peeled and seeded
1½ cups Homemade Chicken Broth
2 tablespoons fresh Parsley, minced
Natural unprocessed Salt, to taste

Directions:
1. Preheat the oven to 400 degrees F and lightly grease a casserole dish.
2. In a large bowl, add the beef, cilantro, mint and garlic, and mix well. Make small balls from the beef mixture.
3. Place the squash pieces in the prepared casserole dish. Pour in the broth and place the meatballs on top. Bake for about 45 minutes.
4. Meanwhile, in a small bowl, mix together the parsley and salt. Remove the casserole from oven once cooked and immediately sprinkle with the salted parsley.

Rosemary Chicken Casserole

This delicious chicken casserole dish will become a popular recipe for entertaining guests and family. This scrumptious dish is also ideal for the winter months.

Servings: 4
Prep Time: 15 minutes
Cooking Time: 2 hours

Ingredients:

3 cups fresh Green Beans, trimmed and sliced
4 Carrots, peeled and sliced
1 large Onion, diced
1 pound cubed, boneless, Organic Chicken Breasts
1½ cups Homemade Chicken Broth
2 tablespoons fresh Rosemary, minced
2 tablespoons fresh Sage, minced
Natural unprocessed Salt, to taste

Directions:

1. Preheat the oven to 300 degrees F and lightly grease a casserole dish.
2. Place the beans, carrots and onion in the prepared casserole dish. Top with the chicken. Pour the broth over the vegetables and chicken.
3. Sprinkle with the fresh herbs and salt. Bake for approximately 2 hours.

Holiday Sprout Casserole

This dish is a wonderful way to cook Brussels sprouts. This casserole is a delightful accompaniment to any holiday meal.

Servings: 4
Prep Time: 15 minutes
Cooking Time: 45 minutes

Ingredients:

20-24 Brussels Sprouts, trimmed, outer leaves removed and halved
2 Onions, quartered
3 Garlic Cloves, sliced lengthwise
1 sprig fresh Thyme
Natural unprocessed Salt, to taste
1 tablespoon Ghee, melted
3 tablespoons Homemade Chicken Broth

Directions:

1. Preheat the oven to 400 degrees F and lightly grease a casserole dish.
2. In a large bowl, toss together all of the ingredients, except for the broth. Transfer the mixture into the prepared casserole dish and add the broth.
3. Cover with foil and bake for 35 to 45 minutes.

Vegetable Medley Casserole

This dish has a bright and colorful combination of vegetables. This casserole is good enough to steal the limelight from your favorite main dishes.

Servings: 4
Prep Time: 15 minutes
Cooking Time: 1 hour 30 minutes

Ingredients:

4 small Zucchinis, peeled, seeded and sliced into ½-inch sections
2 medium Eggplants, cubed
4 Plum Tomatoes, seeded and sliced
2 medium Onions, sliced
1 tablespoon fresh Marjoram, chopped
1 tablespoon fresh Rosemary, chopped
Natural unprocessed Salt, to taste
2 tablespoons Ghee, melted
2 tablespoons Homemade Chicken Broth

Directions:

1. Preheat the oven to 325 degrees F and lightly grease a casserole dish.
2. In a large bowl, add all of the ingredients, except for the broth, and gently toss together. Transfer the mixture into the prepared casserole dish and add the broth.
3. Bake for about 1½ hours.

Fermented Mackerel

This is a great way of fermentation which brings a delicious taste to the fish! It is also a great source of thyroid nutrition.

Servings: 4
Prep Time: 3 - 5 days

Ingredients:

4 fresh skinless, boneless Mackerel, cut into bite size pieces
½ small White Onion, sliced
10 Bay Leaves
1 teaspoon Black Peppercorns
½ teaspoon Cilantro Seeds
½ teaspoon Dill Seeds
1-4 tablespoons Whey
1 tablespoon natural unprocessed Salt
1 cup filtered Water

Directions:

1. In a sterilized jar, add the mackerel, onion, bay leaves, peppercorns and dill.
2. In a jug, mix together the whey, salt and water. Pour the water mixture in the jar to cover the fish pieces.
3. Cover tightly and keep at room temperature for 3 to 5 days before refrigerating to store.

Fermented Whole Sardines

Fermented fish is rich in vitamins and minerals. It is also exceptionally easy to prepare.

Servings: 4
Prep Time: 3 - 5 days

Ingredients:
6-7 fresh Whole Sardines
1 tablespoon natural unprocessed Salt
1 tablespoon crushed or smashed Black Peppercorn
6-7 Bay Leaves
½ teaspoon fresh Dill, minced
1 cup Whey
Filtered Water, as required

Directions:
1. Scrape off the scales from the fish. Cut the heads and thoroughly clean the bellies. In a wide-faced sterilized jar, apart from the water, add the fish and remaining ingredients.
2. Pour the water to cover the fish completely. Close the lid tightly and then cover the jar with a tea towel.
3. Keep at room temperature for 3 to 5 days, then refrigerate to store.
4. When you are ready to eat the fish, take the meat from the bones, cut into bite-size pieces and serve.

Fermented Squid

Salty fermented squid can be eaten as a side dish that can be kept in your fridge for months. You will enjoy this squid until you've eaten the last bite.

Servings: 4
Prep Time: 1 month

Ingredients:
1½ pounds small Squid
4 tablespoons natural unprocessed Salt

Directions:
1. Cut off the tentacles in front of the eyes. Discard the eye parts. Then remove the inner parts and bones. Place the cleaned squid flesh in a bowl. Scrub the squids with your hands. Rinse in cold water and drain completely.
2. Place the squids into a sterilized jar. Sprinkle with salt. Press it down to minimize exposure to the air. Close the lid and refrigerate for 1 month.

Fermented Salmon

This is a great recipe for lacto-fermented fish, which calls for a salmon filet, whey, honey and a few basic herbs and spices.

Servings: 4
Prep Time: 1day

Ingredients:

1 pound Salmon fillet, skinned and cut into bite sized pieces
2 whole Allspice Corns, crushed
8 Black Peppercorns, crushed
2 Bay Leaves
1 bunch fresh Dill, snipped
2 slices of Lemon, seeded
1 cup Filtered Water
1 tablespoon Honey
⅛ cup uncooked Whey
1 tablespoon natural unprocessed Salt

Directions:

1. In a sterilized jar, add the salmon, allspice corns, black peppercorns, bay leaves, dill and lemon slices.
2. In a jug, mix together the water, honey, whey and salt. Pour the water mixture into the jar to cover the fish pieces.
3. Cover tightly and keep at room temperature for about 1 day. Then refrigerate to store.

Healthy Home-style Ghee

This process is quick and painless, and you will end up with a yummy and healthy cooking fat. Ghee has many uses, a few being for sautéing vegetables or meats, used to drizzle over hot rice or as an ingredient in soups.

Prep Time: 5 minutes
Cooking Time: 13 minutes

Ingredients:

1 pound unsalted Butter, chopped

Directions:

1. In a heavy bottomed pan, melt the butter on a medium-low heat.
2. Reduce the heat to low. Now the butter will form a foam which will soon disappear, then re-appear again. After 7-8 minutes the butter will become brown. Remove from heat and cool slightly.
3. Strain the ghee through a cheesecloth or fine strainer. Store in an airtight container until required.

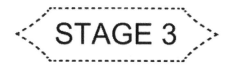

Organic Pumpkin Pancakes

*These pancakes are very easy to prepare, and have an amazing flavor.
These are great for breakfast.*

Servings: 4
Prep Time: 10 minutes
Cooking Time: 4 minutes

Ingredients:

*1 cup Homemade Pumpkin Puree
4 Organic Eggs
Ghee, as required for cooking
Natural unprocessed Salt, to taste*

Directions:

1. In a bowl, beat together the pumpkin puree and eggs.
2. In a frying pan, melt the ghee on a medium-low heat. With a spoon, add the prepared mixture to the pan to make thin pancakes.
3. Cook for 1½ to 2 minutes per side. Repeat with the remaining mixture to make more pancakes.

Coco Squash Pancakes

These pancakes are a wonderfully tasty way to get anyone to eat butternut squash. Enjoy these pancakes as you wish.

Servings: 4
Prep Time: 10 minutes
Cooking Time: 4 minutes

Ingredients:
1 cup cooked, peeled and seeded Butternut Squash
2 Organic Eggs
½ cup Coconut Butter
Ghee, as required for cooking
Natural unprocessed Salt, to taste

Directions:
1. In a food processor, add all of the ingredients, except for the ghee, and pulse until smooth.
2. In a frying pan, melt the ghee on a medium-low heat. With a spoon, add the mixture to the pan to make thin pancakes.
3. Cook for 1½ to 2 minutes per side. Repeat with the remaining mixture to make more pancakes.

Zucchini Master Pancakes

This recipe makes one of the best vegetarian pancakes. These crispy, but light, pan-fried zucchini pancakes make an easy and wonderfully tasty appetizer or side dish.

Servings: 4
Prep Time: 10 minutes
Cooking Time: 4 minutes

Ingredients:

1 large Zucchini, peeled, seeded and cooked
2 Organic Eggs
½ cup Almond Butter
Ghee, as required for cooking
Natural unprocessed Salt, to taste

Directions:

1. In a food processor, add all of the ingredients, except for the ghee, and pulse until smooth.
2. In a frying pan, melt the ghee on a medium-low heat. With a spoon, add the mixture to the pan to make thin pancakes.
3. Cook for 1½ to 2 minutes per side. Repeat with the remaining mixture to make more pancakes.

Almo Pumpkin Pancakes

These pancakes are delicious with butter, and they are perfect for an everyday breakfast.

Servings: 4
Prep Time: 10 minutes
Cooking Time: 4 minutes

Ingredients:

1 cup cooked Pumpkin, peeled and seeded
4 Organic Egg Yolks
½ cup Almond Butter
Ghee, as required for cooking
Natural unprocessed Salt, to taste

Directions:

1. In a food processor, add all of the ingredients, except for the ghee, and pulse until smooth.
2. In a frying pan, melt the ghee on a medium-low heat. With a spoon, add the mixture to the pan to make thin pancakes.
3. Cook for 1½ to 2 minutes per side. Repeat with the remaining mixture to make more pancakes.

Presto Broccoli Pancakes

These festive and beautifully colored pancakes are sure to be a great hit for breakfast.

Servings: 4
Prep Time: 10 minutes
Cooking Time: 4 minutes

Ingredients:
1 cup cooked Broccoli Florets
2 Organic Eggs, egg whites separated
½ cup Coconut Butter
Ghee, as required for cooking
Natural unprocessed Salt, to taste

Directions:
1. In a small bowl, add the egg whites and beat until fluffy.
2. In a food processor, add the beaten egg whites to the remaining ingredients, except for the ghee, and pulse until smooth.
3. In a frying pan, melt the ghee on a low heat. With a spoon, add the mixture to the pan to make thin pancakes.
4. Cook for 1½ to 2 minutes per side. Repeat with the remaining mixture to make more pancakes.

Hearty Carrot Pancakes

These carrot flavored pancakes are hearty and filling enough to be a meal in itself for the whole family.

Servings: 4
Prep Time: 10 minutes
Cooking Time: 4 minutes

Ingredients:
1 cup Carrot, peeled and grated
2 Organic Eggs
½ cup Almond Butter
Ghee, as required for cooking
Natural unprocessed Salt, to taste

Directions:
1. In a pan of boiling water, add the carrot and cook for 4 to 5 minutes. Drain well and transfer onto paper toweling.
2. In a bowl, add the eggs and almond butter, and beat until well combined. Fold in the carrots.
3. In a frying pan, melt the ghee on a medium-low heat. With a spoon, add the mixture to the pan to make thin pancakes.
4. Cook for 1½ to 2 minutes per side. Repeat with the remaining mixture to make more pancakes.

Onion Scrambled Eggs

You may start your morning with this simple, nutritious and great tasting scrambled egg dish.

Servings: 4
Prep Time: 10 minutes
Cooking Time: 5 minutes

Ingredients:

8 Organic Eggs
Ghee, as required for cooking
2 medium Onions, sliced thinly
Natural unprocessed Salt, to taste

Directions:

1. In a bowl, add the eggs and salt, and beat until frothy.
2. In a skillet, melt the ghee on a medium-low heat. Add the onion and sauté for 4 to 5 minutes. Reduce the heat, cover and, whilst stirring occasionally, cook for a further 15 to 20 minutes.
3. Increase the heat to medium. Add the beaten eggs and cook, stirring continuously, for 4 to 5 minutes.

Pumpkin Pleasers Scramble

This dish is very simple to throw together on a weekend. Interestingly, with pumpkin added to the eggs, there is less craving to eat meat.

Servings: 4
Prep Time: 10 minutes
Cooking Time: 5 minutes

Ingredients:
8 Organic Eggs
1 cup Homemade Pumpkin Puree
Ghee, as required for cooking
Natural unprocessed Salt, to taste

Directions:
1. In a bowl, add the eggs and salt, and beat until frothy. Add the pumpkin puree and beat until well combined.
2. In a skillet, melt the ghee on a medium heat.
3. Add the beaten eggs and cook, stirring continuously, for 4 to 5 minutes.

Creamy Avocado Scramble

Even though at first glance, scrambled eggs with avocados might seem weird, this dish is remarkably tasty. This dish is perfect for a light lunch.

Servings: 4
Prep Time: 10 minutes
Cooking Time: 5 minutes

Ingredients:

8 Organic Eggs
Ghee, as required for cooking
1 cup Avocado, peeled, pitted and cut into ½-inch chunks
Natural unprocessed Salt, to taste

Directions:

1. In a bowl, add the eggs and salt, and beat until frothy.
2. In a skillet, melt the ghee on a medium heat.
3. Add the beaten eggs and cook, stirring continuously, for 4 to 5 minutes.
4. Stir in the avocado and immediately remove from heat and serve.

Scrambled Zucchi Eggs

This quick and easy scrambled egg recipe makes a hearty and delicious breakfast for the whole family.

Servings: 4
Prep Time: 10 minutes
Cooking Time: 5 minutes

Ingredients:
8 Organic Eggs
1 large Zucchini, peeled, seeded, cooked and mashed
Ghee, as required for cooking
Natural unprocessed Salt, to taste

Directions:
1. In a bowl, add the eggs and salt, and beat until frothy. Add the mashed zucchini and beat until well combined.
2. In a skillet, melt the ghee on a medium heat.
3. Add the beaten eggs and cook, stirring continuously, for 4 to 5 minutes.

Cauliflower Scramble

Make your breakfast time memorable with this dish of scrambled eggs and mashed cauliflower.

Servings: 4
Prep Time: 10 minutes
Cooking Time: 5 minutes

Ingredients:
8 Organic Eggs
1 cup Cauliflower Florets, cooked and mashed
Ghee, as required for cooking
Natural unprocessed Salt, to taste

Directions:
1. In a bowl, add the eggs and salt, and beat until frothy. Add the mashed cauliflower and beat until well combined.
2. In a skillet, melt the ghee on a medium heat.
3. Add the beaten eggs and cook, stirring continuously, for 4 to 5 minutes.

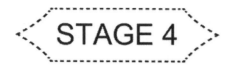

Roasted Chicken Thighs

This is a simple blend of garlic, thyme and seasoning which gives great flavor to these moist chicken thighs. This dish is quickly cooked in the oven and makes a delicious main dish. Serve with cooked carrots.

Servings: 4
Prep Time: 10 minutes
Cooking Time: 1 hour

Ingredients:

2 Garlic Cloves, minced finely
½ teaspoon Dried Thyme, crushed
Natural unprocessed Salt, to taste
Freshly Crushed Black Pepper, to taste
4 (4-ounces each) Organic Chicken Thighs

Directions:

1. Preheat the oven to 350 degrees F and grease a roasting pan.
2. In a large bowl, mix together the garlic, thyme and seasonings. Add the chicken thighs and generously coat with the mixture.
3. Transfer the chicken thighs into the prepared roasting pan and roast for 1 hour.

Herb Roasted Wings

Adding fresh herbs from your garden makes these chicken wings extra special and flavorful. This recipe gives these roasted wings a juicy and moist texture.

Servings: 4
Prep Time: 15 minutes
Cooking Time: 20 minutes

Ingredients:

2 pounds Organic Chicken Wings
1 tablespoon finely diced fresh Thyme Leaves
1 tablespoon finely diced fresh Rosemary Leaves
Natural unprocessed Salt, to taste
Freshly Crushed Black Pepper, to taste

Directions:

1. Preheat the oven to 500 degrees F and line a roasting pan with foil.
2. In a large bowl, add the chicken wings and sprinkle with fresh herbs and seasonings. Mix together to ensure the chicken is thoroughly coated.
3. Arrange the chicken wings in the prepared roasting pan in a single layer. Roast for about 20 minutes, turning once after 10 minutes.

Roasted Lamb Chops

This recipe is a great way to prepare delicious and elegant roasted chops that uses simple flavors. These simply seasoned and roasted lamb chops brilliantly brings out a natural flavor.

Servings: 4
Prep Time: 15 minutes (Plus time to marinate)
Cooking Time: 18 minutes

Ingredients:

1 tablespoon finely diced fresh Rosemary Leaves
1 tablespoon finely diced fresh Oregano Leaves
4 Garlic Cloves, minced
2 tablespoons Unsalted Butter
Natural unprocessed Salt, to taste
Freshly Crushed Black Pepper, to taste
4 (4-ounces each) Organic Lamb Loin Chops

Directions:

1. In a bowl, mix together the fresh herbs, garlic, seasoning and 1 tablespoon of melted butter. Add the chops and generously coat with the marinade. Refrigerate to marinate for at least 1 hour.
2. Preheat the oven to 400 degrees F. In an oven proof skillet, heat the remaining oil on a medium heat. Add the chops and cook for 3 to 4 minutes per side.
3. Transfer the skillet into the oven and roast for 10 minutes.

Buttery Roast Steak

This is an elegant yet simple preparation method for beef tenderloin, cooked in a classic way. This healthy and tasty recipe is perfect for busy nights or holiday meals.

Servings: 4
Prep Time: 10 minutes
Cooking Time: 19 minutes

Ingredients:
1 tablespoon Unsalted Butter
1 pound trimmed Organic Beef Tenderloin Steak
Natural unprocessed Salt, to taste
Freshly Crushed Black Pepper, to taste

Directions:
1. Preheat the oven to 400 degrees F and grease a roasting pan.
2. In a skillet, heat the oil on a medium-high heat. Add the beef to the skillet and sprinkle with salt and black pepper. Cook for about 2 minutes per side.
3. Transfer the beef into the roasting pan. Roast for about 15 minutes, turning once after 8 minutes.

Dilled Roasted Cod

This is a perfect fish for a party meal or weekend family dinner. The secret of this delicious fish is in the garlic mixture which really enhances the flavor.

Servings: 4
Prep Time: 10 minutes
Cooking Time: 15 minutes

Ingredients:

1 tablespoon Garlic, minced
3 tablespoons Ghee, melted
1 tablespoon fresh Dill, minced
Natural unprocessed Salt, to taste
Freshly Crushed Black Pepper, to taste
4 (4-ounces each) Cod Fillets

Directions:

1. Preheat the oven to 400 degrees F and grease a roasting pan.
2. In a small bowl, add all of the ingredients, except the fish, and beat until well combined.
3. Arrange the fillets in the prepared roasting pan, in a single layer. Pour the garlic mixture over the fillets.
4. Bake for 10 to 15 minutes.

Grilled Garlic Lamb

This combination of simple and few ingredients, like fresh herbs and garlic, delivers a fragrant aroma to these lamb chops. This recipe may attract those who don't even like lamb.

Servings: 4
Prep Time: 10 minutes (Plus time to marinate)
Cooking Time: 10 minutes

Ingredients:

3 Garlic Cloves, sliced
1 tablespoon fresh Thyme, minced
1 tablespoon fresh Oregano, minced
2 tablespoons Ghee, melted
Natural unprocessed Salt, to taste
Freshly Crushed Black Pepper, to taste
4 (4-ounces each) Organic Lamb Loin Chops

Directions:

1. In a food processor, add all of the ingredients, except the chops, and pulse until a paste forms. Transfer the mixture into a large bowl. Add the chops and generously coat with the paste. Cover and refrigerate to marinate for at least 1 hour.
2. Remove the chops from refrigerator and sit at room temperature for at least 30 minutes.
3. Preheat the grill to a medium heat. Grease the grill grate. Grill the chops for 4 to 5 minutes per side.

Buttery Garlic Grilled Chicken

This is one of the most tasty and popular dishes for a summer barbeque party. This recipe gives tender, juicy and tasty flavors to the chicken. Garlic infused butter is the main secret to these flavors.

Servings: 4
Prep Time: 15 minutes
Cooking Time: 30 minutes

Ingredients:

2 Garlic Cloves, minced
3 tablespoons melted Unsalted Butter
Natural unprocessed Salt, to taste
Freshly Crushed Black Pepper, to taste
4 (4-ounces each) (bone-in and skin on) Organic Chicken Breast Halves

Directions:

1. In a small bowl, mix together the fresh garlic, melted butter, a pinch of salt and black pepper. Set aside for at least 15 minutes. Meanwhile, sprinkle the chicken with salt and black pepper, and set aside for 10 minutes for the seasoning to infuse.
2. Preheat the grill to its highest setting. Grease the grill grate and place under the heat. Once the grill grate is very hot, turn off the grill.
3. Brush the chicken with the butter and garlic mixture. Place the chicken on the very hot grill grate. Cover and cook for 15 minutes. Turn and cook for 10 minutes more.
4. Turn on the grill again, and grill the chicken for a further 5 minutes on each side.

Grilled Chicken Drumsticks

These grilled chicken legs have a wonderful "kick" from the flavorful marinade of garlic, fresh herbs and butter. This dish is sure to be a crowd pleaser!

Servings: 4
Prep Time: 15 minutes (Plus time to marinade)
Cooking Time: 30 minutes

Ingredients:

1 tablespoon fresh Rosemary, minced
1 tablespoon fresh Thyme, minced
2 Garlic Cloves, minced
1 tablespoon Unsalted Butter, melted
Natural unprocessed Salt, to taste
Freshly Crushed Black Pepper, to taste
8 Organic Chicken Legs

Directions:

1. In a large bowl, add all of the ingredients, except the chicken legs, and beat until well combined. Add the chicken legs and coat with the marinade. Cover and, for at least 24 hours, refrigerate. Turn the chicken legs often.
2. Preheat the grill to a medium-high heat. Grease the grill grate.
3. Grill the chicken legs for 30 minutes. Turn the chicken every 5 minutes.

Grilled Halibut Supreme

This is a superb halibut dish. This grilled fish gets its perfection from its simple but flavorful marinade.

Servings: 4
Prep Time: 10 minutes (Plus time to marinate)
Cooking Time: 10 minutes

Ingredients:

1 teaspoon Dried Thyme, minced
Natural unprocessed Salt, to taste
Freshly Crushed Black Pepper, to taste
1 tablespoon Ghee, melted
4 (4-ounces each) Halibut Fillets

Directions:

1. In a small bowl, add the thyme, salt and black pepper, and mix well. In a large bowl, add the fish fillets and generously coat with the dry mixture. Cover and refrigerate to marinate for at least 1 hour.
2. Preheat the grill to a medium heat. Grease the grill grate.
3. Remove the fish from the marinade and shake off any excess marinade. Brush the fillets with melted ghee.
4. Cook the fish for 5 minutes each side.

Oregano Grilled Steak

The simple marinade in this recipe gives fantastic flavors to each slice of flank steak. This steak will melt in your mouth! Enjoy with steamed broccoli.

Servings: 4
Prep Time: 10 minutes (Plus time to marinate)
Cooking Time: 12 minutes

Ingredients:

1 teaspoon Dried Oregano, minced
1 large Garlic Clove, minced
Natural unprocessed Salt, to taste
Freshly Crushed Black Pepper, to taste
1 pound Organic Flank Steak, trimmed

Directions:

1. In a large bowl, add all the ingredients, except the steak, and mix well. Add the steak and generously coat with the marinade. Cover and refrigerate for at least 3 to 4 hours.
2. Preheat the grill to a medium-high heat. Grease the grill grate.
3. Cook the chops for 5 to 6 minutes per side.

Easy-O Almond Bread

This recipe, being simple and tasty, will provide a delicious bread perfect for breakfast.

Servings: 4
Prep Time: 10 minutes
Cooking Time: 1hour

Ingredients:
½ cup Almond Flour
¼ cup Unsalted Butter, softened
3 Organic Eggs, beaten
Pinch of Natural unprocessed Salt

Directions:
1. Preheat the oven to 300 degrees F and grease a loaf pan.
2. In a bowl, add all the ingredients and beat until well combined. Transfer the mixture into the prepared loaf pan.
3. Bake for about 1 hour, or until a toothpick inserted into the center comes out clean.

Pecan & Onion Bread

This is a savory bread with a combination of eggs and pecans. Ground pecans add a slightly nutty crunch to this uniquely flavored bread.

Servings: 4
Prep Time: 15 minutes
Cooking Time: 1hour 20 minutes

Ingredients:
¼ cup plus 1 teaspoon softened Unsalted Butter
2½ cups Crispy Pecan Nuts
3 Organic Eggs, beaten

Directions:
1. Preheat the oven to 300 degrees F and grease a loaf pan.
2. In a frying pan, heat the softened butter on a medium heat. In a food processor, add the pecans and pulse until finely ground. Transfer the ground pecans into the bowl with softened butter and mix well.
3. In another bowl, add the egg which is the remaining ingredient and beat until well combined. Add the pecan and butter mixture and mix. Transfer the mixture into the prepared loaf pan.
4. Bake for about 1 hour, or until a toothpick inserted into the center comes out clean.

Winter Almond Bread

This easy bread recipe is perfect for those who love the flavor of squash. It will be great for lunch boxes and anytime snacks.

Servings: 4
Prep Time: 15 minutes
Cooking Time: 1hour 20 minutes

Ingredients:
4 cups Almond Flour
¼ cup Unsalted Butter, softened
4 Organic Eggs, beaten
1 cup Winter Squash, peeled, seeded, cooked and mashed
Pinch of Natural unprocessed Salt

Directions:
1. Preheat the oven to 300 degrees F and grease a loaf pan.
2. Transfer the almond flour into a bowl.
3. In another bowl, add the remaining ingredients, and beat until well combined. Mix in the almond flour. Add 1-2 more eggs if the mixture appears too dry or a little more almond flour if the mixture appears too wet. Transfer the mixture into the prepared loaf pan.
4. Bake for about 80 minutes, or until a toothpick inserted into the center comes out clean.

Nutty Carrot Bread

This is a tasty bread infused with the flavors of almonds and cooked carrots.

Servings: 4
Prep Time: 15 minutes
Cooking Time: 1 hour 20 minutes

Ingredients:
4 cups Almond Flour
¼ cup Ghee, softened
4 Organic Eggs, beaten
1 cup Carrots, peeled, cooked and mashed
Pinch of Natural unprocessed Salt

Directions:
1. Preheat the oven to 300 degrees F and grease a loaf pan.
2. In a food processor, add the almonds and pulse until finely ground. Transfer the ground almonds into a bowl.
3. In another bowl, add the remaining ingredients and beat until well combined. Mix in the ground almonds. Transfer the mixture into the prepared loaf pan.
4. Bake for about 80 minutes, or until a toothpick inserted into the center comes out clean.

Nut-Free Zucchini Bread

This is a nut-free bread for those who want to avoid nuts. This simple recipe makes crispy thin bread which will be great for sandwiches.

Servings: 4
Prep Time: 15 minutes
Cooking Time: 40 minutes

Ingredients:
4 Organic Egg Yolks
⅓ cup Zucchini, peeled, seeded, cooked and mashed
6 Organic Egg Whites
Pinch of Natural unprocessed Salt

Directions:
1. Preheat the oven to 300 degrees F. Line a glass Pyrex dish with greased parchment paper.
2. In a bowl, add the egg yolks and zucchini, and beat until well combined. In another bowl, add the egg whites and salt, and beat until soft peaks form. Fold the egg yolk mixture into the egg white mixture. Transfer the mixture into the prepared Pyrex dish.
3. Bake for about 30 minutes, or until a toothpick inserted into the center comes out clean. Remove from the oven. With a flat spatula, gently remove the bread from the dish. Remove the parchment paper.
4. Return the bread into the dish, bottom side up. Bake for a further 10 minutes.

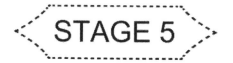

Grilled Spinado Chicken

This grilled chicken with fresh spinach and avocadoes makes a wonderfully nutritious main course meal for the whole family.

Servings: *4*
Prep Time: *15 minutes (Plus time to marinate)*
Cooking Time: *10 minutes*

Ingredients:

- For Chicken -
2 Garlic Cloves, minced finely
3 teaspoons fresh Thyme, minced
1 tablespoon Unsalted Butter, melted
Natural unprocessed Salt, to taste
Freshly Crushed Black Pepper, to taste
2 (4-ounces each) skinless, boneless Organic Chicken Breasts

- For Vegetables -
4 cups fresh Baby Spinach Leaves
4 Ripe Avocados, peeled, pitted and sliced
2 tablespoons finely diced fresh Mint Leaves
2 tablespoons Extra Virgin Olive Oil
Natural unprocessed Salt, to taste
Freshly Crushed Black Pepper, to taste

Directions:

1. For the chicken, in a large bowl add all of the ingredients and toss to coat well. Cover and refrigerate to marinate

for about 30 minutes.

2. Preheat the grill to a high heat and grease the grill grate. Cook the chicken for 4 to 5 minutes per side. Let the breasts sit for 5 minutes before cutting the breasts into thin slices.

3. Meanwhile, in a large serving bowl, place the spinach, avocado and mint leaves. Top with the chicken pieces.

4. Drizzle with olive oil and sprinkle with salt and pepper. Toss to coat well before serving.

Grilled Flank Steak

This is one of those recipes which is created with a minimum of fuss. This grilled steak with fresh vegetables is just fantastic for a barbeque party.

Servings: 4
Prep Time: 20 minutes
Cooking Time: 10 minutes

Ingredients:

- For Flank Steak -
10-ounces Organic Flank Steak, trimmed
Natural unprocessed Salt, to taste
Freshly Crushed Black Pepper, to taste

- For Vegetables -
¼ cup Red Onion, chopped
¼ cup Scallions, sliced thinly
½ cup diced English Cucumber, peeled and seeded
1 cup Cherry Tomatoes, halved
2 tablespoons Extra Virgin Olive Oil
Natural unprocessed Salt, to taste
Freshly Crushed Black Pepper, to taste
2 cups Butter Lettuce, torn

Directions:
1. Preheat the grill to a high heat and grease the grill grate. Generously sprinkle the steak with salt and black pepper. Grill the steak for 4 to 5 minutes per side. Let the steak sit for 10 minutes before cutting into ½-inch slices.
2. Meanwhile, in a large bowl, mix together the onion, scallion, cucumber and tomatoes. Drizzle with oil and sprinkle with salt and black pepper. Toss to coat well. Set

aside.

3. For serving, in a large serving bowl, place torn lettuce. Place the vegetables over the lettuce. Top with steak slices and serve.

Grilled Tuna Salad

Grilled tuna is one of the most popular and versatile fishes. In this recipe the fish pairs nicely with the salad of carrots and red onion.

Servings: 4
Prep Time: 20 minutes (Plus time to marinate)
Cooking Time: 10 minutes

Ingredients:

- *For Tuna* -
2 Garlic Cloves, minced
1 tablespoon finely diced fresh Rosemary Leaves
Natural unprocessed Salt, to taste
Freshly Crushed Black Pepper, to taste
2 (6-ounces) fresh Tuna Steaks
1 teaspoon Unsalted Butter, melted

- *For Vegetables* -
½ cup Red Onion, sliced thinly
1½ cups Cucumber, peeled, seeded and cut into matchsticks
1½ cups Carrots, peeled and cut into matchsticks
1 tablespoon Extra Virgin Olive Oil
Natural unprocessed Salt, to taste
Freshly Crushed Black Pepper, to taste

Directions:

1. In a bowl, mix together the garlic, rosemary, salt and black pepper. Add the tuna steaks and coat with the marinade, set aside to marinate for at least 20 minutes.
2. Preheat the grill to a high heat and lightly grease the grill grate. Brush the steaks with melted butter. Cook the steaks for 3 minutes per side before cutting the steaks into bite sized pieces.

3. Meanwhile, in a large bowl, mix together the onion, cucumber and carrots. Drizzle with oil and sprinkle with salt and black pepper. Toss to coat well. Set aside.

4. For serving, in a large serving bowl, place the vegetables. Top with the tuna steak pieced and serve immediately.

Crunchy Eggs Salad

Welcome spring by combining hard boiled eggs with a crunchy mixture of fresh baby spinach, carrot, cabbage and grape tomatoes.

Servings: 4
Prep Time: 20 minutes

Ingredients:

3 cups fresh Baby Spinach
½ cup Carrot, peeled and shredded
½ cup Cabbage, shredded
½ cup Grape Tomatoes, halved
3 Hard Boiled Eggs, diced
2 tablespoons Extra Virgin Olive Oil
Natural unprocessed Salt, to taste
Freshly Crushed Black Pepper, to taste

Directions:

1. In a large bowl, mix together the spinach, carrot, cabbage, tomatoes and eggs.
2. In another bowl, combine together the oil, salt and black pepper.
3. Pour the dressing over the salad and toss well.

Shades of Green Salad

This is a nutritionally balanced and satisfying salad which is fresh and crunchy.

Servings: 4
Prep Time: 20 minutes

Ingredients:

1 Cucumber, peeled, seeded and chopped
½ cup Broccoli Florets, chopped finely
4 Scallions, chopped
1½ cups chopped fresh Romaine Lettuce
1½ cups Cabbage, grated
½ cup fresh Basil Leaves, chopped
3 tablespoons Extra Virgin Olive Oil
Natural unprocessed Salt, to taste
Freshly Crushed Black Pepper, to taste

Directions:

1. In a large bowl, add all of the ingredients and toss well.
2. Serve immediately.

Herbed Vegetable Salad

This healthy fresh salad of cucumbers, onion and tomatoes is accompanied with fresh herbs. This salad may be a great hit if served with some grilled meat.

Servings: 4
Prep Time: 20 minutes

Ingredients:

1 cup Cucumber, peeled, seeded and chopped
1 cup Red Onion, sliced thinly
2 cups Cherry Tomatoes, halved
½ cup fresh Parsley Leaves, chopped
¼ cup fresh Mint leaves, chopped
3 tablespoons Extra Virgin Olive Oil
Natural unprocessed Salt, to taste
Freshly Crushed Black Pepper, to taste

Directions:

1. In a bowl mix together the cucumber, onion, tomatoes, parsley and mint.
2. In another bowl, mix together the remaining ingredients.
3. Pour the dressing over the salad and toss well before serving.

Minty Beet Salad

This is a beautifully red colored salad with a refreshing green hint from the mint. It is also very delicious and appetizing. Garnish with extra mint leaves.

Servings: 4
Prep Time: 20 minutes

Ingredients:

2 cups Carrots, peeled and grated
2 cups Beetroots, peeled and grated
2 Scallions, sliced thinly
2 tablespoons finely diced fresh Mint Leaves
3 tablespoons Extra Virgin Olive Oil
Natural unprocessed Salt, to taste
Freshly Crushed Black Pepper, to taste

Directions:

1. In a large bowl, mix together all of the ingredients.
2. Serve immediately.

Zucchini Meatball Casserole

This meatball casserole is great as a flavorful dinner. Grated zucchini gives the beef meatballs a wonderful boost, and keeps them moist. Garnish with chopped fresh basil or cilantro leaves.

Servings: 4
Prep Time: 15 minutes
Cooking Time: 35 minutes

Ingredients:
2 tablespoons Ghee
2 Garlic Cloves, minced
1 Red Onion, shredded
5 small Zucchinis, peeled, seeded and shredded
Natural unprocessed Salt, to taste
Freshly Crushed Black Pepper, to taste
1½ cups tomatoes, peeled, seeded and chopped finely
1 pound Organic Lean Ground Beef
1 Organic Egg, beaten
1 tablespoon fresh Cilantro, minced
1 tablespoon fresh Mint, minced

Directions:
1. Preheat the oven to 350 degrees F.
2. In a large oven proof skillet, melt the ghee on a medium heat. Sauté the garlic for 30 seconds. Add the onion and zucchini, and sprinkle with salt and black pepper. Sauté for 2 to 3 minutes. Add the tomatoes and cook, stirring, for 2 minutes. Remove from the heat.
3. In a bowl mix together the beef, egg, fresh herbs, salt and black pepper. Make small sized balls from the mixture.
4. Place the balls in the skillet, gently pressing down into the vegetable mixture. Transfer the skillet into the oven and bake for 25 to 30 minutes.

Roasted Chicken Broccoli

This classic combination of chicken and broccoli makes a delicious and hearty dish. This super easy recipe is a great hit for a family dinner. Serve with a freshly made salad.

Servings: 4
Prep Time: 15 minutes
Cooking Time: 45 minutes

Ingredients:

4 (4-ounces each) boneless, skinless Chicken Thighs (Organic)
6 cups Broccoli Florets
3 tablespoons Ghee, melted
1 teaspoon Dried Thyme, crushed
Natural unprocessed Salt, to taste
Freshly Crushed Black Pepper, to taste

Directions:

1. Preheat the oven to 375 degrees F and lightly grease a baking dish.
2. Place the chicken and broccoli in the prepared dish. Drizzle with the melted ghee and sprinkle with thyme, black pepper and salt.
3. Roast for about 45 minutes.

Carrot Chicken Stew

This is one of the easy, but super delicious chicken stews. The chicken breast makes a perfect combination with baby carrots. Garnish with chopped fresh parsley.

Servings: 4
Prep Time: 15 minutes
Cooking Time: 1 hour 45 minutes

Ingredients:

2 tablespoons Ghee, melted
1 Onion, chopped
2 Garlic Cloves, minced
2 Celery Stalks, chopped
4 (4-ounces each) diced boneless, skinless Chicken Breast Halves (Organic)
½ cup tomatoes, peeled, seeded and chopped finely
1½ pounds Baby Carrots, trimmed
1 cup Homemade Chicken Broth
Natural unprocessed Salt, to taste
Freshly Crushed Black Pepper, to taste

Directions:

1. In a large soup pan, melt the ghee on a medium heat. Sauté the onion, garlic and celery for 4 to 5 minutes.
2. Add the chicken and cook for a further 4 to 5 minutes. Add the tomatoes and cook for an additional 4 to 5 minutes, crushing the tomatoes whilst cooking.
3. Add the carrots and broth, and bring to the boil. Reduce the heat and, whilst covered, simmer for 1 to 1½ hours.
4. Season with salt and black pepper and serve hot.

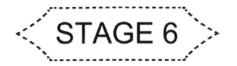

Haz-o-nut Cake

This easy recipe makes a great teatime cake which is simply delicious.

Servings: 4
Prep Time: 10 minutes
Cooking Time: 35 minutes

Ingredients:

⅔ *cup Hazelnut Meal*
6 Organic Eggs
¼ *cup Unsalted Butter*

Directions:

1. Preheat the oven to 338 degrees F and grease a cake tin.
2. In a food processor, add all of the ingredients and pulse until smooth. Place the mixture in the cake tin.
3. Bake for 25 to 35 minutes, or until done.

Peanut Butter Raisin Cake

This nourishing peanut butter and pecan cake is addictive. What makes this cake extra special is that it does not need to be baked! It will make a great snack or a treat.

Servings: 4
Prep Time: 10 minutes

Ingredients:
2 cups Crispy Pecans
½ cup natural Peanut Butter, softened
½ cup Coconut Oil, melted
⅓ cup Raisins
½ teaspoon natural unprocessed Salt

Directions:
1. Grease a cake tin.
2. In a food processor, add the pecans and pulse until coarsely chopped. Add the remaining ingredients then pulse until smooth.
3. Place the mixture in the cake tin. Refrigerate until it has set completely.

Banana Peak Pancakes

Pump up the flavor of your homemade pancakes with peanut butter and banana. These will quickly become a favorite combination for your family.

Servings: 4
Prep Time: 10 minutes
Cooking Time: 4 minutes

Ingredients:
3 Organic Eggs, beaten
2 tablespoons softened Salted Peanut Butter
1 Ripe Banana, peeled and mashed
Ghee, as required for cooking

Directions:
1. In a large bowl, beat together all of the ingredients.
2. In a frying pan, melt the ghee on a medium-low heat. With a spoon, add enough mixture to the pan to make a thin pancake.
3. Cook for 1½ to 2 minutes per side. Repeat with the remaining mixture to make more pancakes.

Squash & Zucchini Pancakes

These squash and zucchini pancakes will go a long way for lunch or breakfast. By combining these simple ingredients you will end up with pancakes that even kids will love.

Servings: 4
Prep Time: 10 minutes
Cooking Time: 4 minutes

Ingredients:
1 cup Almond Meal
2 Organic Eggs, beaten
⅓ cup cooked Butternut Squash, peeled, seeded and pureed
⅓ cup cooked Zucchini, seeded, peeled and pureed
Pinch of natural unprocessed Salt
Ghee, as required for cooking

Directions:
1. In a large bowl, beat together all of the ingredients.
2. In a frying pan, melt the ghee on a medium-low heat. With a spoon, add enough mixture to the pan to make a thin pancake.
3. Cook for 2 to 3 minutes per side. Repeat with the remaining mixture to make more pancakes.

Flourless Squash Muffins

These savory squash muffins are great for anyone who eats a gluten-free and grain-free diet. The squash gives these muffins a beautiful lemony color.

Servings: 4
Prep Time: 10 minutes
Cooking Time: 40 minutes

Ingredients:
4 Organic Eggs, separated
1 tablespoon Unsalted Butter
1½ cups cooked Yellow Squash, peeled, seeded and pureed
Pinch of natural unprocessed Salt

Directions:
1. Preheat the oven to 300 degrees F and grease a small muffin tray.
2. In a bowl, add the egg whites and beat until soft peaks form.
3. In a food processor, add the egg yolks and remaining ingredients, and pulse until smooth. Stir in the egg whites.
4. Place the mixture in the muffin tray. Bake for 30 to 40 minutes, or until a toothpick inserted into the center comes out clean.

Almond Banana Muffins

These light muffins are ideal for a healthy and delicious breakfast, as well for an afternoon snack. These muffins are also a great way to use up ripe bananas.

Servings: 4
Prep Time: 10 minutes
Cooking Time: 50 minutes

Ingredients:
2½ cups Almond Flour, sifted
3 Organic Eggs, beaten
¼ cup Unsalted Butter, softened
2 Ripe Bananas, peeled and pureed

Directions:
1. Preheat the oven to 300 degrees F and grease a large muffin tray.
2. In a large bowl, mix together all of the ingredients.
3. Place the mixture into the muffin tray. Bake for about 50 minutes, or until a toothpick inserted into the center comes out clean.

Zucchini Almond Muffins

Zucchini is especially wonderful for adding moisture to these delicious muffins. These muffins can be enjoyed all winter long!

Servings: 4
Prep Time: 10 minutes
Cooking Time: 30 minutes

Ingredients:
2 cups Almond Flour, sifted
6 Organic Eggs, beaten
¼ cup Unsalted Butter, softened
2 cups Zucchini, peeled, seeded and grated
Pinch of natural unprocessed Salt

Directions:
1. Preheat the oven to 350 degrees F and grease a muffin tray.
2. In a food processor, add all of the ingredients and pulse until smooth. Place the mixture into the prepared muffin tray.
3. Bake for 20 to 30 minutes, or until a toothpick inserted into the center comes out clean.

Pumpkin Pecan Muffins

This is a nice recipe to make light and airy muffins. These pumpkin muffins are full of nutritional value and loaded with wonderful flavors.

Servings: 4
Prep Time: 10 minutes
Cooking Time: 30 minutes

Ingredients:
2 cups Pecan Flour, sifted
6 Organic Eggs, beaten
¼ cup Ghee, melted
2 cups cooked Pumpkin, peeled, seeded and pureed
Pinch of natural unprocessed Salt

Directions:
1. Preheat the oven to 350 degrees F and grease a muffin tray.
2. In a food processor, add all of the ingredients and pulse until smooth. Place the mixture into the muffin tray.
3. Bake for 20 to 30 minutes, or until a toothpick inserted into the center comes out clean.

Baked Veggie Meatballs

These baked lamb meatballs are the perfect dish for the lamb lover. These meatballs offer a wonderful combination with a simple grilled vegetable medley.

Servings: 4
Prep Time: 20 minutes
Cooking Time: 20 minutes

Ingredients:

- For Meatballs -

1¼ pounds Organic Ground Lamb
1 small Organic Egg, beaten
2 tablespoons finely diced fresh Cilantro Leaves
Natural unprocessed Salt, to taste
Freshly Crushed Black Pepper, to taste

- For Veggies -

1 small Onion, chopped
2 Garlic Cloves, minced
2 small Summer Squashes, seeded, peeled and sliced
2 small Zucchinis, seeded, peeled and sliced
1 Tomato, seeded and diced
1 tablespoon Ghee, melted
1 teaspoon Dried Thyme, crushed
Natural unprocessed Salt, to taste
Freshly Crushed Black Pepper, to taste

Directions:

1. Preheat the oven to 350 degrees F and line a baking pan with foil. In a large bowl, mix together all of the meatball ingredients. Make your desired sized balls with the meat mixture. Place the meatballs in the prepared baking dish

and bake for 20 minutes.

2. Meanwhile, preheat the grill to a medium heat and line the grill pan with foil. Place the onion and garlic in the pan. Spread the squash, zucchini and tomatoes over the onion and garlic then drizzle with the melted ghee. Sprinkle with thyme, salt and black pepper.

3. Fold the foil paper and seal tightly. Place the grill pan under the grill and cook for 15 to 20 minutes.

4. On a serving plate, serve the grilled vegetables with the baked meatballs.

Beef & Squash Bake

This delicious baked dish is hearty and full of protein and flavors. This recipe is a great way to use up the bounty of squash in the garden, and is also guaranteed to leave no empty bellies.

Servings: 4
Prep Time: 15 minutes
Cooking Time: 50 minutes

Ingredients:

1 pound Organic Lean Ground Beef
1 small Acorn Squash, peeled, seeded and cubed
1 small Butternut Squash, cubed, seeded and peeled
1 small cubed Yellow Squash, peeled and seeded
1 teaspoon Dried Rosemary, crushed
1 teaspoon Dried Thyme, crushed
Natural unprocessed Salt, to taste
Freshly Crushed Black Pepper, to taste
1 tablespoon Ghee, melted

Directions:

1. Preheat the oven to 400 degrees F and grease a baking dish.
2. In the prepared baking dish add all of the ingredients and mix well. Drizzle with the melted ghee.
3. Cover with foil and bake for 30 minutes. Remove the foil and stir the beef and squash mixture. Bake, uncovered, for an additional 20 to 30 minutes.

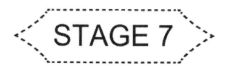

STAGE 7

If you have managed to reach this stage of the diet. Congratulations! You have successfully reached the full stage recipes. Enjoy these recipes and experience the benefits of completing the diet fully. Be reminded that you may continue to use recipes from all previous stages.

BREAKFAST RECIPES

Beef Scrambled Eggs

By combining beef, mushrooms and onion make this simple scrambled egg dish extra hearty for a special breakfast.

Servings: 4
Prep Time: 15 minutes
Cooking Time: 15 minutes

Ingredients:
2 tablespoons Ghee
½ Onion, chopped finely
¾ pound Organic Ground Beef
1 cup Mushrooms, chopped
8 Organic Eggs
Natural unprocessed Salt, to taste
Freshly Crushed Black Pepper, to taste
1 Avocado, pitted and chopped

Directions:
1. In a skillet, heat the oil on a medium heat. Sauté the

onion for 2 minutes. Add the beef and cook for 2 to 3 minutes. Add the mushrooms and, whilst stirring, cook for 4 to 5 minutes.

2. In a bowl, beat together the eggs, salt and black pepper. Pour the egg mixture into the skillet. Cook, stirring continuously, for 4 to 5 minutes.

3. Place the scrambled eggs on a serving plate and top with avocado.

Eggs & Zucchini Fiesta

This simple summer egg skillet, made with zucchini and scallion, is not only healthy, but makes a super tasty breakfast meal as well.

Servings: 4
Prep Time: 15 minutes
Cooking Time: 25 minutes

Ingredients:
2 tablespoons Ghee
1 medium White Onion, chopped
1 Scallion, chopped
4 cups Zucchinis, peeled, seeded and diced
Natural unprocessed Salt, to taste
4 Organic Eggs
Freshly Crushed Black Pepper, to taste

Directions:
1. In a skillet heat the oil on a medium-low heat. Sauté the onion and scallion for 6 to 8 minutes. Add the zucchini and sauté for 6 to 7 minutes, then stir in the salt.
2. Make four wells in the vegetable mixture at equal distances. Reduce the heat to low. Carefully crack the eggs into each well.
3. Cover and cook for 5 to 10 minutes. Sprinkle with black pepper before serving.

Poached Egg Salad

Poaching is one of the simplest and easiest ways to prepare an egg. This fresh salad, topped with poached eggs, is perfect as a satisfying breakfast or brunch, or even for a light lunch.

Servings: 4
Prep Time: 15 minutes
Cooking Time: 5 minutes

Ingredients:

- For Salad -
4 cups torn Romaine Lettuce Leaves
2 Cucumbers, peeled, seeded and chopped
1 Avocado, pitted and sliced
1 teaspoon Extra Virgin Olive Oil

- For Poached Eggs -
1 teaspoon White Vinegar
Natural unprocessed Salt, to taste
8 Organic Eggs
Freshly Crushed Black Pepper, to taste

Directions:

1. Divide the lettuce onto 4 serving plates. Evenly top with the cucumber and avocado. Drizzle with oil and set aside.
2. To a pan of boiling water, add the vinegar and salt. Reduce the heat to medium-low. Crack an egg into a cup then carefully add the egg into the simmering water. Using a spoon, keep the egg white close to the yolk. Turn off the heat. Cover tightly and set aside for 5 minutes. Repeat with the remaining eggs.
3. Place 2 poached eggs onto each plate, on top of the salad.

STAGE 7
Sprinkle with salt and black pepper before serving.

Cheesy Sausage Bake

This is a hearty meal for Sunday mornings. Eggs, cheese, sausage and spinach mingle in this crowd-pleasing bake very nicely.

Servings: 4
Prep Time: 15 minutes
Cooking Time: 56 minutes

Ingredients:
2 tablespoons Unsalted Butter
1 small Onion, chopped
½ pound (diet friendly) Ground Sausage
1 Garlic Clove, minced
1 cup Cooked Chicken, shredded
½ cup Spinach, chopped
½ cup Swiss Cheese, cubed
1 cup Cheddar Cheese, cubed
8 Organic Eggs
Natural unprocessed Salt, to taste
Freshly Crushed Black Pepper, to taste

Directions:
1. Preheat the oven to 350 degrees F and grease a small baking dish.
2. In a skillet, melt the butter on a medium heat. Add the onion and sausage and cook for 4 to 5 minutes before adding the garlic and cooking for an additional minute. Transfer the sausage mixture into the prepared baking dish. Combine the chicken, spinach and cheese into the baking dish.
3. In a bowl, beat together the eggs, salt and black pepper. Evenly pour the egg mixture over the mixture in the baking dish.
4. Bake for 40 to 50 minutes.

Honey Crepes

These super quick almond flour crepes whip up a nutritious breakfast within a minute. These crepes are simple to make and slightly sweetened with a mild honey flavor.

Servings: 4
Prep Time: 10 minutes (Plus time to refrigerate)
Cooking Time: 1 minute

Ingredients:
5 Organic Eggs
2 teaspoons Organic Honey
½ cup plus 2 tablespoons Blanched Almond Flour
Pinch of natural unprocessed Salt
2 tablespoons Filtered Water
Melted Butter, as required for cooking

Directions:
1. In a bowl, beat together the eggs and honey.
2. In another bowl, mix together the flour and salt. Add the egg mixture and beat until all lumps are removed. Add the water and mix until smooth and creamy. Cover and refrigerate for 15 minutes.
3. Grease a cast iron pan with melted butter and heat on a medium heat. Add ¼ cup of batter into the pan. Swirl the batter around the pan to spread it evenly. Cook for about 45 seconds. Gently flip and cook for 10 to 15 seconds.
4. Repeat with the remaining batter. Transfer the cooked crepes onto a serving plate.

Honey Almond Pancake

Combine all of the ingredients together and bake for a quick and delicious pancake breakfast. This is an easy dish for a big family, and less time consuming than making individual pancakes.

Servings: 4
Prep Time: 10 minutes
Cooking Time: 25 minutes

Ingredients:
¼ cup Unsalted Butter
6 Organic Eggs
1 cup Homemade Yogurt
1 teaspoon Organic Honey
1 cup Almond Flour
¼ teaspoon natural unprocessed Salt

Directions:
1. Preheat the oven to 425 degrees F, and butter a 13x9-inch baking dish. Place the dish into the oven to melt the butter.
2. In a bowl, beat together the eggs, yogurt and honey. In another bowl, combine the flour and salt. Mix the egg mixture into the flour mixture.
3. After the butter is melted, pour the batter into the dish. Bake for about 25 minutes.
4. Cut into desired sizes and serve.

Cinapple Muffins

You can kick-start your morning with these delicious apple muffins. These muffins, made with a pinch of cinnamon, have a wonderful aromatic smell that will encourage you to make them time and time again.

Servings: 4
Prep Time: 10 minutes
Cooking Time: 22 minutes

Ingredients:
3 Organic Eggs, separated
3 tablespoons Organic Honey
2 tablespoons melted Unsalted Butter
¼ cup Coconut Flour, sifted
1 teaspoon Ground Cinnamon
¼ teaspoon natural unprocessed Salt
1 Apple, peeled, cored and diced

Directions:
1. Preheat the oven to 350 degrees F and grease a 12 cup muffin tray.
2. In a bowl, beat the egg whites until soft peaks form. In a second bowl, add the egg yolks, honey and butter, and beat well. In a third bowl, combine the cinnamon and flour with the salt.
3. Mix the egg yolk mixture into the flour mixture. Fold in the diced apple and egg whites. Place the mixture into the prepared muffin tray.
4. Bake for 20 to 22 minutes, or until a toothpick inserted into the center comes out clean.

Cocobana Bread

This recipe makes a classic, moist and delicious bread packed with banana flavor. Your whole family, especially your kids, will love to eat this delicious bread.

Servings: 4
Prep Time: 10 minutes
Cooking Time: 1 hour

Ingredients:
6 tablespoons Coconut Flour, sifted
½ teaspoon Ground Cinnamon
¼ teaspoon natural unprocessed Salt
3 Organic Eggs
¼ cup Organic Honey
2 tablespoons melted Unsalted Butter
1 small Ripe Banana, peeled and mashed

Directions:
1. Preheat the oven to 325 degrees F and grease a small 7.5x3.75-inch loaf pan.
2. In a bowl, mix together the flour, cinnamon and salt. In another bowl, beat together the eggs, honey, butter and banana.
3. Mix the egg mixture into the flour mixture. Place the mixture in the prepared loaf pan.
4. Bake for 50 to 60 minutes, or until a toothpick inserted into the center comes out clean.

LUNCH RECIPES

Nutty Fish Salad

This is a perfect salad made with fish, crisp asparagus and crunchy walnuts, with a mustard dressing. This quick and healthy salad is great for an elegant lunch in spring.

Servings: 4
Prep Time: 15 minutes
Cooking Time: 5 minutes

Ingredients:

- *For Dressing* -
1 tablespoon fresh Lemon Juice
2 tablespoons Extra Virgin Olive Oil
1 teaspoon Mustard Powder
Natural unprocessed Salt, to taste
Freshly Crushed Black Pepper, to taste

- *For Salad* -
½ pound fresh Asparagus, trimmed and cut into 1-inch pieces
½ cup Grilled Herring, cut into 1-inch chunks
½ cup cooked Green Peas
2 Heads Romaine Lettuce, torn
¼ cup Walnuts, toasted and chopped
2 Hard Boiled Eggs, peeled and sliced

Directions:

1. In a pan of boiling water, add the asparagus and cook for 5 minutes before draining.
2. In a bowl, mix together the lemon juice, oil, mustard, salt and black pepper.

3. In a large serving bowl, add all of the remaining ingredients, except for the eggs, and mix together. Pour over the dressing and toss to coat well.
4. Top with egg slices and serve.

Green Lentil Soup

This is a winter soup with layers of flavors. Fresh kale, lime and a thyme sprig brighten up the flavor of these lentils for a warm, nutritious and hearty soup.

Servings: 4
Prep Time: 15 minutes
Cooking Time: 30 minutes

Ingredients:
6 cups Homemade Chicken Broth
1½ cups Green Lentils, rinsed
1 sprig fresh Oregano
2 tablespoons Unsalted Butter
1 large Onion, chopped
2 Garlic Cloves, minced
½ teaspoon Ground Cinnamon
Pinch of Ground Nutmeg
1 cup Kale, trimmed and chopped
1 cup unsweetened Coconut Milk
1 tablespoon fresh Lime Juice
Natural unprocessed Salt, to taste
Freshly Crushed Black Pepper, to taste

Directions:
1. In a large soup pan, add the broth, lentils and oregano, and bring to the boil on a high heat. Reduce the heat to medium-low, cover and simmer for 20 minutes. Discard the oregano sprig.
2. Meanwhile, in a skillet, melt the butter on a medium heat. Sauté the onion for 12 to 15 minutes, or until caramelized. Add the garlic, cinnamon and nutmeg, and sauté for 30 seconds. Transfer the onion mixture into the pan with the lentils.

3. Stir in the kale and coconut milk. Cook for 10 minute more.

4. Stir in the lime juice, salt and black pepper before serving.

Cauliflower Baked Chicken

This high-protein baked dish of chicken, cauliflower and olives is great for a wonderful lunch. This dish is a hit with adults and teens alike.

Servings: 4
Prep Time: 15 minutes (Plus time to marinate)
Cooking Time: 1 hour

Ingredients:

1 tablespoon Ghee, melted
2 tablespoons fresh Lime Juice
1 teaspoon Lime Zest, grated freshly
1 small Onion, chopped
2 Garlic Cloves, minced
Natural unprocessed Salt, to taste
Freshly Crushed Black Pepper, to taste
1 fresh Rosemary Sprig
1½ pounds Organic Chicken Legs
1 cup Cauliflower Florets
½ cup Black Olives, pitted and sliced

Directions:

1. In a bowl, mix together the ghee, lime juice, zest, onion, garlic, salt and black pepper. Set aside.
2. In a baking dish, place the rosemary sprig, and place the chicken legs on top. Place the cauliflower florets and olives over the chicken legs. Finally, pour the ghee mixture over the chicken and vegetables before covering and refrigerating overnight.
3. Preheat the oven to 400 degrees F and bake for about 1 hour.

Lamb & Bean in Coconut Sauce

This nice and simple recipe makes the lamb especially tender and aromatic. This is one of the best and most delicious meals for all!

Servings: 4
Prep Time: 15 minutes
Cooking Time: 37 minutes

Ingredients:
1½ tablespoons Ghee
½ pound Organic Lamb, cut into bite sized pieces
1 Onion, chopped
2 Garlic Cloves, minced
1 cup Broccoli florets
1½ cups Tomatoes, peeled and chopped finely
Natural unprocessed Salt, to taste
Freshly Crushed Black Pepper, to taste
¼ teaspoon Cayenne Pepper
4 cups Homemade Chicken Broth
1¼ cups cooked White Beans
1 Bay Leaf
1¼ cups Coconut Milk
1 tablespoon fresh Parsley, chopped

Directions:
1. In a large skillet melt the ghee on a medium heat. Add the lamb and cook for 4 to 5 minutes. Transfer the lamb onto a plate. In the same skillet sauté the onion for 4 to 5 minutes. Add the garlic and sauté for 1 minute more.
2. Add the broccoli, tomatoes, salt, black pepper and cayenne pepper, and cook for 3 to 4 minutes. Add the lamb, broth, beans and bay leaf, and bring to boiling point.

110

3. Reduce the heat to medium-low. Cover and simmer for 15 to 20 minutes. Add the parsley and coconut milk, and continue cooking for a further 2 minutes.
4. Serve hot.

Cheesy Portobello Mushrooms

These stuffed Portobello mushrooms are easy to put together and have a beautiful presentation. This dish is perfect for guests at lunch times, as well as making a great combination with a steak or a giant salad.

Servings: 4
Prep Time: 15 minutes
Cooking Time: 15 minutes

Ingredients:

4 Portobello Mushroom Caps
Natural unprocessed Salt, to taste
Freshly Crushed Black Pepper, to taste
4 teaspoons Extra Virgin Olive Oil
2 tablespoons Balsamic Vinegar (without sugar)
2 Garlic Cloves, minced
¼ cup cooked Chicken, shredded finely
4 Artichoke Hearts, sliced finely
4 cups fresh Baby Spinach Leaves
1 tablespoon fresh Thyme Leaves
¼ cup Feta Cheese, crumbled

Directions:

1. Preheat the oven to 400 degrees F and grease a baking sheet. Place the mushroom caps on the prepared baking sheet. Sprinkle with black pepper and salt, and drizzle with 2 tablespoons of oil and vinegar.
2. In a skillet, heat the remaining oil on a medium heat. Sauté the garlic for 1 minute. Add the chicken, artichoke and spinach, and cook for 3 to 4 minutes. Season with salt and black pepper.
3. Remove from the heat and immediately stir in the thyme

and cheese. Evenly fill each mushroom cap with the stuffing.

4. Place the mushroom caps onto the prepared baking sheet and bake for 10 minutes.

Yogurt Turkey Meatballs

This dish of ground turkey meatballs with mint yogurt sauce is quick and easy to make. This recipe creates delicious and flavorful meatballs.

Servings: 4
Prep Time: 15 minutes
Cooking Time: 25 minutes

Ingredients:

1 pound Organic Ground Turkey
½ teaspoon Garlic, minced finely
½ Onion, chopped
¼ cup fresh Parsley Leaves, chopped
1 tablespoon fresh Lemon Juice
1 cup Homemade Yogurt, divided
¼ teaspoon Ground Cinnamon
Pinch of Cayenne Pepper
Natural unprocessed Salt, to taste
Freshly Crushed Black Pepper, to taste
½ teaspoon fresh Mint Leaves, minced

Directions:

1. Preheat the oven to 400 degrees F and grease a baking dish.
2. In a large bowl, combine the turkey, garlic, onion, parsley, lemon juice, 3 tablespoons of yogurt, cinnamon, cayenne pepper, salt and black pepper. Make your desired sized balls from the mixture. Place the balls in the prepared baking dish and bake for 25 minutes, turning once after 13 minutes.
3. In a bowl, mix together the remaining yogurt, mint and a pinch of salt and black pepper.
4. Pour the sauce over meatballs and serve.

Peppery Broccoli Steak

This delicious stir fry can be prepped without any fuss. The ginger gives a nice sweet heat to this meal, and the broccoli gives it a beautiful and bright color.

Servings: 4
Prep Time: 15 minutes (Plus time to marinate)
Cooking Time: 10 minutes

Ingredients:

- For Beef Marinade -
1 tablespoon fresh Ginger, grated finely
¼ cup Homemade Chicken Broth
2 tablespoons Cider Vinegar
1 tablespoon Organic Honey
Natural unprocessed Salt, to taste
Freshly Crushed Black Pepper, to taste
¼ teaspoon Cayenne Pepper
½ teaspoon Ground Cumin
1 pound Sirloin Steak, cut into thin strips

- For Stir Fry -
2 tablespoons Ghee
2 Garlic Cloves, minced
1-inch fresh Ginger Piece, sliced very thinly
1 cup small Broccoli Florets
¼ cup fresh Cilantro, chopped

Directions:
1. In a large bowl, mix together all of the marinade ingredients, except for the beef. Add the beef and generously coat with the marinade before covering and refrigerating for 24 hours.

2. In a skillet, melt the ghee on a medium-high heat. Remove the beef from the marinade and reserve the marinade. Add the beef into the skillet and cook for 2 to 3 minutes. Transfer the beef onto a plate and pour the reserved marinade over the beef.
3. In the same skillet, sauté the ginger and garlic in the ghee for 1 minute. Add the broccoli and stir fry for 3 to 4 minutes.
4. Stir in the beef with the marinade and stir fry for a further 2 minutes. Top with cilantro and serve.

Creamy Baked Cod

This recipe ensures a tender, succulent and flavorful fish. The sauce, made with coconut milk and parsley, nicely enhances the delicate and wonderful flavors of the fish.

Servings: 4
Prep Time: 15 minutes (Plus time to marinate)
Cooking Time: 10 minutes

Ingredients:

½ teaspoon Garlic, minced finely
½ tablespoon Fresh Ginger, minced finely
1 tablespoon Organic Honey
1½ cups Coconut Milk
¼ teaspoon Ground Cinnamon
½ teaspoon Ground Cumin
Natural unprocessed Salt, to taste
Freshly Crushed Black Pepper, to taste
1 pound Cod Fillets
2 tablespoons fresh Parsley, chopped

Directions:

1. In a large bowl, combine all of the ingredients, except for the cod. Add the cod and generously coat with the marinade before covering and refrigerating for 30 minutes.
2. Preheat the oven to 400 degrees F and grease a baking dish.
3. Remove the cod from marinade, reserve the marinade. Place the fish fillets in the prepared baking dish and top with parsley. Bake for 12 to 18 minutes. Meanwhile, in a pan, add the reserved marinade and bring to boiling point on a medium heat. Cook the marinade for a further 2 minutes.

4. Pour the marinade sauce over the cod before serving.

DINNER RECIPES

Zesty Turkey Salad

With this recipe, tender slices of turkey, with flavorful tomatoes and cucumber, are served over a bed of spinach which makes this a truly fabulous and tasty salad for lunch.

Servings: 4
Prep Time: 15 minutes

Ingredients:

- *For Dressing* -
1½ tablespoons fresh Lemon Juice
2 teaspoons Lemon Zest, grated freshly
2 tablespoons Extra Virgin Olive Oil
Natural unprocessed Salt, to taste
Freshly Crushed Black Pepper, to taste

- *For Salad* -
2 cups cooked Organic Turkey, chopped
1½ cups halved Red Cherry Tomatoes
1½ cups halved Yellow Cherry Tomatoes
1 large Cucumber, peeled and chopped
¼ cup Red Onion, chopped
2 tablespoons Scallions, sliced thinly
2 tablespoons fresh Basil Leaves
¼ cup fresh Parsley Leaves, chopped
¼ cup Feta Cheese, crumbled
Baby Spinach Leaves, as required

Directions:
1. In a bowl, mix together the lemon juice, zest, oil, salt and black pepper.

2. In a large serving bowl, mix together all of the salad ingredients, except for the cheese. Pour the dressing onto the salad and toss.

3. Place the spinach leaves on serving plates and place the salad on top. Top with the cheese and serve.

Roasted Vegetable Soup

Roasted vegetables cooked with broth, spinach and lima beans make up this hearty and yummy soup.

Servings: 4
Prep Time: 15 minutes
Cooking Time: 60 minutes

Ingredients:

1 large Onion, cut into 8 wedges
5 whole Garlic Cloves, unpeeled
2 large Tomatoes, quartered
1 small Zucchini, peeled, seeded and cut into thick wedges
½ small Butternut Squash, seeded and cut into thick wedges
2 medium Carrots, peeled and quartered lengthwise
1 tablespoon Extra Virgin Olive Oil
Natural unprocessed Salt, to taste
Freshly Crushed Black Pepper, to taste
6 cups Homemade Chicken Broth
2 fresh Oregano Sprigs
3 cups fresh Spinach, torn
1 Bay Leaf
1½ cups cooked Lima Beans

Directions:

1. Preheat the oven to 400 degrees F and grease a rimmed baking sheet. Place the vegetables on the prepared baking dish. Drizzle with oil and sprinkle with salt and black pepper before roasting for 45 minutes.
2. In a food processor, puree together the onion, peeled garlic and tomatoes. Cut the roasted zucchini, squash and carrots into ½-inch pieces.
3. In a large soup pan, add the pureed tomato mixture, broth, oregano and bay leaf. Bring to a boil on a high

heat. Reduce the heat to low and simmer for 25 minutes.
4. Add the zucchini, squash, carrot, spinach and beans. Simmer for 15 minutes more, then season with salt and black pepper before serving.

Lamb Deal

This recipe is an easy way to prepare roast lamb chops with vegetables. These tasty, succulent lamb chops make the perfect midweek dinner which is full of delicious flavors.

Servings: 4
Prep Time: 15 minutes
Cooking Time: 40 minutes

Ingredients:

1 large Onion, cut into wedges
1 large Zucchini, peeled, seeded and cut into wedges
1 large Yellow Squash, seeded and cut into wedges
1 Red Bell Pepper, seeded and cut into chunks
1 Green Bell Pepper, seeded and cut into chunks
1 Orange Bell Pepper, seeded and cut into chunks
Natural unprocessed Salt, to taste
Freshly Crushed Black Pepper, to taste
1 tablespoon Ghee, melted
8 Organic Lean Lamb Chops
2 tablespoons finely diced fresh Rosemary Leaves
1 tablespoon finely diced fresh Thyme Leaves

Directions:

1. Preheat the oven to 425 degrees F and line a roasting pan. Place the onion, zucchini, squash and bell peppers in the prepared roasting pan. Sprinkle with black pepper and salt, and drizzle with the melted ghee. Roast for 20 minutes.

2. Meanwhile, in a bowl mix together the salt, black pepper, rosemary and thyme. Add the chops and generously coat with mixture.

3. Remove the roasting pan from the oven. Push the vegetables to the side and add the chops to the pan. Bake

for 20 minutes, turning the chops after 10 minutes.
4. Serve the chops with the vegetables.

Baked Beef Casserole

This fantastic and easy to prepared casserole dish is layered with beef and fresh vegetables. This one-pot meal is great for family potlucks.

Servings: 4
Prep Time: 15 minutes
Cooking Time: 6 hours

Ingredients:
1 pound Organic Beef Stew Meat
3 large Carrots, peeled and cut into chunks
2 cups Tomatoes, chopped
1 medium Onion, chopped
1 stalk Celery, chopped
¼ teaspoon fresh Rosemary, minced
¼ teaspoon fresh Marjoram, minced
¼ teaspoon fresh Thyme, minced
Natural unprocessed Salt, to taste
Freshly Crushed Black Pepper, to taste
¼ cup Red Wine

Directions:
1. Preheat the oven to 250 degrees F.
2. In a casserole dish, place all of the ingredients and mix well.
3. Cover and bake for 5 to 6 hours, occasionally stirring.

Carrot Baked Chicken

This easily prepared succulent baked chicken is perfect when entertaining many people.

Servings: 4
Prep Time: 15 minutes
Cooking Time: 40 minutes

Ingredients:

1 large Onion, cut into bite size pieces
1 stalk Celery, cut into bite size pieces
3 Carrots, peeled and cut into bite size pieces
1 cup small Broccoli Florets
1 tablespoon White Vinegar
2 tablespoons Extra Virgin Olive Oil
Natural unprocessed Salt, to taste
Freshly Crushed Black Pepper, to taste
½ teaspoon Dried Thyme, crushed
½ teaspoon Dried Oregano, crushed
1 pound Organic Chicken Thighs

Directions:

1. Preheat the oven to 425 degrees F and lightly grease a baking dish.
2. Place all of the vegetables in the prepared pan. Drizzle with vinegar and half of the oil. Sprinkle with salt, black pepper and herbs.
3. Brush the chicken with the remaining oil, and sprinkle with black pepper and salt. Arrange the chicken thighs over the vegetables and bake for 1 hour. Transfer the chicken onto a plate and cover with foil to keep warm.
4. Mix together the vegetables and bake for a further 5 to 10 minutes. Serve the chicken with the vegetables.

Gingery Zucchini Lamb

This authentic lamb stew with zucchini and spices is perfect for a family dinner. The zucchini and ginger lightens the flavor of the lamb, perfectly.

Servings: 4
Prep Time: 15 minutes
Cooking Time: 2 hours 32 minutes

Ingredients:

2 tablespoons Ghee
1 pound Organic Lamb Stew Meat
Natural unprocessed Salt, to taste
Freshly Crushed Black Pepper, to taste
1 Yellow Onion, chopped
2 stalks Celery, chopped
¼ teaspoon fresh Ginger, minced
¼ teaspoon Cayenne pepper
1 Garlic Clove, minced
1 teaspoon ground Cumin
2 cup Tomatoes, peeled and chopped
1 cup Homemade Chicken Broth
¼ cup fresh Cilantro, chopped
2 small Zucchinis, peeled, seeded and chopped
1 Organic Egg
1 tablespoon fresh Lemon Juice
2 tablespoons finely diced fresh Mint Leaves

Directions:

1. In a large pan, melt the ghee on a medium-high heat. Add the lamb and sprinkle with black pepper and salt. Cook, stirring continuously, for 4 to 5 minutes. Add the onion and celery and sauté for 3 to 4 minutes. Add the garlic, ginger, cayenne pepper and cumin, and sauté for a further minute.

2. Add the tomatoes and cook, stirring occasionally, for about 10 minutes. Add the broth and cilantro, and bring to a boil. Reduce the heat to low, cover and simmer for about 2 hours. Stir in the zucchini and simmer for a further 10 minutes.

3. In a bowl beat together the egg and lemon juice. Pour this mixture into the pan and stir gently. Cover and cook for 1 to 2 minutes.

4. Season with salt and black pepper then serve, topped with fresh mint leaves.

Honey Spiced Baked Salmon

This is one of the most enjoyable and easily baked fish dishes. This fantastic, healthy and delicious recipe is bursting with flavors of olives, honey and spices.

Servings: 4
Prep Time: 15 minutes (Plus time to marinate)
Cooking Time: 51 minutes

Ingredients:

2 tablespoons fresh Lemon Juice
Natural unprocessed Salt, to taste
Freshly Crushed Black Pepper, to taste
1 teaspoon Dried Rosemary, crushed
1 pound Salmon Fillets
1½ tablespoons Ghee
½ cup Onion, chopped
¼ teaspoon fresh Ginger, minced
1 Garlic Clove, minced
¼ teaspoon Ground Cumin
¼ teaspoon Ground Cilantro
2 cups Tomatoes, chopped finely
½ tablespoon Organic honey
2 tablespoons Black Olives, pitted and sliced
2 tablespoons Green Olives, pitted and sliced
2 tablespoons fresh Parsley, chopped

Directions:

1. Add the fish to a bowl and drizzle with 1 tablespoon of lemon juice. Sprinkle with salt, pepper and rosemary, cover, and refrigerate to marinate for 30 minutes.
2. Preheat the oven to 350 degrees F and lightly grease a baking dish.
3. In a skillet, melt the ghee on a medium heat. Sauté the onion for 4 to 5 minutes. Add the garlic, ginger, cumin

and cilantro, and sauté for a further minute. Add the tomatoes and cook, stirring occasionally, for 10 minutes. Stir in the olives, the remaining lemon juice, and the honey. Cook for an additional 5 minutes.

4. Place the fish fillets in the prepared baking dish and pour over the olive mixture. Sprinkle with salt, black pepper and parsley, and bake for 20 to 30 minutes.

Lamb & Bean Stew

This stew is filled with the superb richness of lamb and vegetables. Mushrooms and beans also give this dish an earthy dimension.

Servings: 4
Prep Time: 15 minutes
Cooking Time: 1hr 27minutes

Ingredients:

2 tablespoons Ghee
1 pound Organic Lamb Stew Meat
Natural unprocessed Salt, to taste
Freshly Crushed Black Pepper, to taste
1 medium Onion, chopped
2 cups Grape Tomatoes, chopped
½ cup fresh Mushrooms, sliced
1 teaspoon Dried Thyme, crushed
½ cup White Wine
½ cup Homemade Chicken Broth
1 cup fresh Green Beans, trimmed and cut into 2-inch pieces

Directions:

1. In a large pan, melt the ghee on a medium-high heat. Add the lamb and sprinkle with black pepper and salt. Cook, stirring continuously, for 4 to 5 minutes.
2. Add the onion and sauté for 5 minutes. Add the tomatoes, mushrooms and thyme, and cook, stirring occasionally, for a further 5 minutes. Add the wine and cook for 2 minutes more.
3. Add the broth and bring to a boil. Simmer, covered, on a low heat for 1 hour.
4. Stir in the green beans and simmer for a further 10 minutes. Season with salt and black pepper before serving.

Yoggie Baked Beef

This delicious and comforting baked dish is packed with flavorful and tender beef. The yogurt and spices adds a unique flavor to this dish.

Servings: 4
Prep Time: 15 minutes
Cooking Time: 1 hour 55 minutes

Ingredients:
3 tablespoons Ghee
1 pound Organic Beef Stew, cubed
Natural unprocessed Salt, to taste
Freshly Crushed Black Pepper, to taste
1 large Onion, chopped
¼ teaspoon fresh Ginger, minced
3 Garlic Cloves, minced
½ tablespoon Paprika
¼ teaspoon Cayenne Pepper
1 cup Homemade Yogurt, beaten

Directions:
1. Preheat the oven to 350 degrees F.
2. In an oven proof casserole pan, melt the ghee on a medium-high heat. Add the beef and sprinkle with black pepper and salt. Cook, stirring continuously, for 4 to 5 minutes. Transfer the beef onto a plate.
3. In the same pan sauté the onion for 8 to 9 minutes. Add the ginger, garlic, paprika and cayenne pepper, and sauté for 1 minute more. Add the yogurt and bring to a gentle simmer, and return the beef to the pan. Wrap tightly with a foil then cover with the lid.
4. Bake for 1 hour 40 minutes.

Herbed Halibut Stew

Fish lovers will fall for this flavorful stew featuring halibut, ginger, wine and parsley. You will find this combination of ingredients to be absolutely unforgettable.

Servings: 4
Prep Time: 15 minutes
Cooking Time: 25 minutes

Ingredients:

3 tablespoons Ghee
1 cup Onion, chopped
¼ teaspoon fresh Ginger, minced
3 Garlic Cloves, minced
1 large Tomato, seeded and chopped finely
¼ cup fresh Parsley Leaves, chopped
½ cup Dry White Wine
1 cup Homemade Fish Broth
1¼ pounds Halibut Fillets, cut into 2-inch pieces
Natural unprocessed Salt, to taste
Freshly Crushed Black Pepper, to taste
¼ teaspoon Dried Thyme, crushed

Directions:

1. In a large skillet, melt the ghee on a medium-high heat. Sauté the onion for 4 minutes. Add the garlic and ginger sauté for 1 minute more.
2. Add the tomatoes and parsley and, whilst stirring occasionally, cook for 10 minutes.
3. Add the fish, wine and broth, and bring to a boil. Simmer, covered, on a medium-low heat for 8 to 10 minutes.
4. Stir in salt, black pepper and thyme before serving.

JUST DO IT!

As you may agree, success in anything starts with equipping yourself with the right tools and information and then applying the principles all the way through. If you'll stick to the *GAPS Diet*, living free from digestive related disorders or a leaky gut is quite an attainable goal. With all the recipes in this cookbook, you are already headed towards achieving that goal.

Additionally, with the simple ingredients and directions in this cookbook, you will be able to successfully create healthy and flavorful gut-friendly meals that will support a healthy gut and lifestyle—and that in itself is simply marvelous.

Thank you for choosing my cookbook. If you find this book to be helpful, I would appreciate if you would let other readers know about it by leaving a book review. I hereby wish you all the best on your quest to experience restored health through a healthy gut. Recover with GAPS!

Best of health,
Pamela Jenkins

Made in the USA
Lexington, KY
27 February 2015